TEDDY BEAR'S TRIUMPH:

TALES FROM A

MEDICAL ALLOTMENT

Harvey Sagar

Published by Harvey Sagar

Copyright © 2013 Harvey Sagar

All rights reserved.

ISBN: 978-0-9575537-0-5

Contents

Preface

Chapter 1: Sowing the seed

Chapter 2: Germination

Chapter 3: Growth

Chapter 4: Nurturing

Chapter 5: Blossoming

Chapter 6: Inspection

Chapter 7: Foreign varieties

Chapter 8: Fruition

Chapter 9: Pesticides, nutrients & other health-giving chemicals

Chapter 10: Legal requirements

Chapter 11: Postscript

Preface

This book is based upon a true story. Only the names, places, circumstances and events have been changed in order to protect the innocent.

Throughout this book, I refers to me and them refers to everyone else. The rest is open to interpretation.

Unattributed quotations are by the author but have not yet been quoted. Quotations attributed to Bob Dylan are by Bob Dylan. The others are self-explanatory.

Medicine is the only profession that labours incessantly to destroy the reason for its own existence.   James Bryce

I'm not really a career person. I'm a gardener, basically. George Harrison

Chapter 1: Sowing the seed

A seed is essentially a plant in a very small box.

I blame my mother. And my teddy bear. Well not really, but without those two I wouldn't be writing this book because I wouldn't have studied medicine and this book is about medicine.

My mother was physically on the short side (or height-disadvantaged as I believe we say these days). She was five feet two inches in her stockinged feet. I cannot say what she was in her non-stockinged feet because she would never be seen in such a state of undress. She was aware that height does not dictate other qualities: diamonds are not made as big as bricks, as she informed a teasing lofty neighbour. She had ambition, and I have to say heart, far exceeding her physical frame. I suspect she got her ambition from her father, whom I never knew. Although not rich, he had no hesitation in buying her a piano to fulfil her desire (sadly never achieved) of becoming a concert pianist. He showed Victorian-style encouragement, wanting to know, for example, why my mother did not come first in the class when she told him she came second. Women in those days (she was born in 1914) were never likely to achieve as much as men professionally because of the social constraints so I suspect that she transferred her ambition onto the men around her. I don't think this was confined to me. She certainly told my father on many occasions that he could achieve more than he did although perhaps she did not put it quite so politely.

At first sight, Teddy seemed healthy enough but he was not a well bear. Like an indulgent father, I attended to his every complaint with thorough attention to detail and a desire to do whatever was in my power to help. Thus, Teddy was at the heart of my first forays into surgery. Instruments in those days were limited to a blunt penknife but, despite the technical limitations and the lack of anaesthetic, I managed to carry out a number of what I would regard as successful operations in pursuit of Teddy's complaints. As I discovered to be a surgical maxim later in life, the operation went well but the patient failed to recover. Despite an assiduous search through his internal straw, I could never find any pathology to account for his symptoms. In order to oblige, I would regularly remove some of the straw to show him postoperatively that treatment had been carried out but he would only come back with more complaints requiring more surgery. After a while, Teddy was embroidered from head to hind paw with incisions, carefully sutured using my mother's darning needle and wool. It was only later that I heard of Munchausen's syndrome, which is a condition where people feign illness in order to attract attention. I realised then that that diagnosis summed up my teddy bear.

My aunt was also complicit in the choose-a-career-for-the-child conspiracy. She was even shorter than my mother but, unlike her, did not have the strength of character to compensate for her physical limitations. She had once been a psychiatric nurse but I suspect this was so she could get access to a ward before she became a full-time patient, as she later did. She moved into working in a television and wireless shop but her short career in nursing seemed to give her unqualified authority to opine on all matters medical. Quite why she changed from nursing to electrical retail is unclear but it may have had something to do with the owner with whom she developed a fixation. I doubt that the feelings were reciprocated but, if they were, it probably says more about the mental health of Mr. Fisher, the proprietor, given the poverty of physical or mental attraction in my aunt. He did once buy her a string of pearls, though.

My aunt lived with my grandmother not far away from us and we would visit every Sunday. From my father's perspective, I am sure this was for the sake of my grandmother because, in respect of my aunt, he couldn't stand her. However, whatever the reasons, the weekly visit left me exposed to the combined influences of my mother and aunt and, since I usually took him with me, my psychologically disadvantaged teddy bear as well.

And so the scene was set. Each phase of growing up was geared around a future career in medicine. Not that I didn't have fun as a child or even that my mother and aunt didn't encourage me to have a happy and fulfilling childhood and adolescence – it was just that there was an implicit understanding that the happiness and fulfilment were self-evidently being experienced by a future doctor.

We worry about what a child will become tomorrow, yet we forget that he is someone today. Stacia Tauscher

The education establishment was also clearly complicit in this plot. After all, it is a lot easier to steer a child along the route necessary to achieve his or her expressed goal than to identify the goal as well as doing the steering. To be fair, the issue of career choice never really came up until there was a need to choose A-level subjects. Until then, the expectation was simply to "do your best" whatever was put in front of you.

Knowing that I was going to be a doctor, I realised how important it was to "get on". Fortunately, the 50s and 60s were highly meritocratic. Success was rewarded handsomely and failure was either scorned or ignored. At primary school, recognition took the form of being to made to stand on one's chair if successful at gaining ten out of ten in a test, not by way of some form of deviant punishment but so that the rest of the class could gaze in awe at this paragon of intellectual virtue. At my grammar school, parents received "fortnightly lists" which detailed their darling offspring's position in class at each subject. The average position across all subjects was reflected in the seating position in class, the better performers being nearer the teacher. It always struck me that it would have been better the other way round because presumably the worst performers were in need of the most attention but nobody else seemed to have thought of it. By the way, fortnightly lists were issued once a month.

My mother loved the system, provided it conformed to her possibly biased assessment of her son's abilities. She had only two reactions to my academic performance: delight at my high positions in class and disdain for my assessors if my position was low. I don't recall my teddy bear's having an opinion.

Have you ever been in therapy? No? You should try it. It's like a really easy game show where the correct answer to every question is: 'Because of my mother.' Robin Greenspan

When the time came to move from primary to secondary school, those considered "suitable" were encouraged to apply for one of the direct grant schools because, frankly, their results were better. I applied for Manchester Grammar School, Bury Grammar School and William Hulme's Grammar School. My mother's reaction to my success at gaining places at Manchester Grammar School and Bury Grammar School but not William Hulme's was to march down to the latter school to enquire with some vigour why her son had been excluded when lesser worthies had been accepted. I can only assume that the psychological beating inflicted on the recipient of this enquiry by my mother produced some acute confusional state because he changed his mind and accepted me, probably contrary to all the rules. So with a place at William Hulme's now assured, I went to Manchester Grammar School, or MGS.

Until then, the furthest I had ever travelled was on holiday. Most of the time we went to Southport, partly, I suspect, because my parents' deep-seated traditionalism would not allow them to break with the Victorian establishment of a seaside resort for Manchester (Mancunians don't count Liverpool) but also to a large extent because my mad aunt was almost as much in love with Lord Street, arguably the most prestigious street in Southport, as she was with her employer. If I had known then that Napoleon lived on that street for a couple of years in the mid-nineteenth century, and had told her, we may have had more varied holidays because she hated the French (almost as much as the Germans) even though, to the best of my knowledge, she had never met any. Anyway, the journey from home to school seemed about as far as the trip to Southport: a ten-minute walk to the bus stop; wait for the bus (which fortunately in those days came every ten minutes and on time); four-mile trip into Cannon Street, stopping, it seemed to me, about every hundred yards; ten-minute walk across central Manchester; and a four-mile bus trip to school. At least one of these bus journeys was better on the way back because I was asleep. I didn't seem to come to much harm even when I came home on the number fifty-nine bus instead of the sixty and, as a result, in winter had to walk in complete darkness along a cinder track down the side of a mill. Maybe paedophilia is a recent invention.

After several years at the school, we had progressed to holidaying in Devon, which may have been responsible for the broadening of my horizons, assisted no doubt by escalating levels of testosterone. The journey to school became SO much within the capabilities of male teenagers like me and my friends. So much so that we made a party of it, usually by stopping off at the Cona coffee bar in Tib Lane to see Judie and have coffee served by her from one of those round glass jugs that sit on a heating element until the coffee has developed the colour of molasses and the taste of quinine. Sometimes we had apple pie as well and, later in our Cona career, cigarettes. I managed to visit the Cona every single schoolday for a whole term.

I suspect a lot more was going on in the Cona than passed our dawning adolescent awareness. The most decadent experience for me was getting in the way of Bubbles Beverley as I was sitting in front of the juke box she wanted to access. As she leant across me, her breasts, which we in the medical profession call large, seemed to embrace my face. For some reason, she found the task easier by placing her hand on the inside of my thigh and asking if I was feeling sexy (darling). I cannot imagine that a schoolboy in uniform had the qualities necessary to prompt this as a serious question, unless she had specialised tastes.   In any case, judging by a previous encounter of hers related to Judie in which she drew a parallel between part of the man's physique and a tenpin bowling skittle, I felt not up to the task. I was also not very keen on catching something.

At MGS, we were blessed with a teacher who held responsibility for careers guidance and a dedicated careers room.   Unfortunately, the careers teacher never seemed available, at least to discuss careers, and the careers room bore a startling resemblance to one of those stands in a hotel foyer, containing a mismatch of unrelated leaflets tempting the passerby to sample some new adventure, visit a garden or have a fun-for-all-the-family day, often at great expense.   The careers teacher and careers room also functioned independently of each other, at least in so far as he was never in it. Thus, it became very difficult to get an opinion on how to choose between Ancient Greek and accounting, should one need to. Needless to say, non-mainstream and non-academic careers didn't get a look in. If you were one of the forward-looking pupils (or their parents) who had formulated their career prior to entering secondary school, so much the better, especially if it was law, medicine or divinity. Rest assured no-one would dream of disrupting such a good plan.

The school was so successful academically that it could afford to pick and choose from the educational rewards on offer. For most students, entry to the sixth form was taken for granted so O-levels (now known as GCSEs) became, for the school, just a burdensome necessity along the way. The number of O-level subjects taken by most of us was therefore limited to four, the minimum requirement for moving on to the "real" qualifications, the A-levels. Seeking unnecessary academic rewards was deemed rather vulgar. What on earth would an MGS student DO with ten O-levels, for goodness sake? Some of us were allowed to take pure maths, as well as maths, at O-level but our later request to take pure maths with statistics A-level on the grounds that the pure maths part was covered in the O-level and the statistics part in an option we had taken in the sixth form was dismissed as an attempt at "badge collecting". I would still quite like the badge, actually.

The real focus on medicine started around the time of entry to the sixth form and choice of A-level subjects simply because it was difficult to defer commitment any longer. Until then, life within and without school was fairly ordinary, at least by the standards of a teenager in the 60s. Many better accounts have been given of life in the 60s than is possible here but suffice it to say that the only changes noticeable from previous decades that I remember were the explosive emergence of modern pop music by The Beatles et al., the protest movement of Bob Dylan et al., sexual freedom, long hair and, above all, short dresses. Apparently there were drugs as well.

The miniskirt was, of course, pioneered by Jean Shrimpton but a study of the photographs of That Dress now seems to show that it was really rather long. It may have been a shock to society, especially the parents within it, when it first appeared but, like many shocking happenings, proved to be only a foretaste of more dramatic things to come. The hemline moved progressively upwards until the only decent way for a male to speak to a young female was when both were standing; him sitting and her standing or him standing and her sitting provided far too much visual information. That did not seem to worry a cameraman on Top of the Pops, however, who adopted a low camera angle to record the gyrations of the dancing teeny guests on the show, all of whom seemed to be female. The broadcast movie sequence looked like a fashion shoot for Marks and Spencer lingerie. His artistry did a great deal to enhance my gender awareness.

I can say without fear of contradiction that I discovered both The Beatles and Bob Dylan, the former in my bedroom and the latter in Lewis's department store in central Manchester. One evening, I was lying on the bedroom floor, listening to Radio Luxembourg whilst simultaneously trying to achieve nirvana with the aid of a book on hatha yoga I had borrowed from the Reference Library in St. Peter's Square, when I heard the now familiar refrain of "Love Me Do" bursting from the transistor radio. Immediately recognising this as progressive music, I listened carefully for the names of the artists when the song had finished because I had a deep sense of the potentially greatest contribution to the musical arts since Schubert. Not long after my revolutionary insight, The Beatles were famous.

My first LP was "In the Wind" by Peter, Paul and Mary, a thoroughly pleasant folk trio who, it seemed to me, perhaps in the error of youth, never did or sang anything very controversial. Even "Blowing in the Wind", the words of which address directly the prejudices and uncaring attitude of society, was sung with a sweetness similar to that of "Lavender's Blue".

> *Lavender's blue, dilly, dilly; lavender's green.*
> *When I am king, dilly, dilly, you shall be queen.*
> *Call up your men, dilly, dilly; set them to work,*
> *Some to the plough, dilly, dilly; some to the fork;*
> *Some to make hay, dilly, dilly; some to cut corn,*
> *While you and I, dilly, dilly, keep ourselves warm.*

But I loved it. I loved it, that is, until one day on my return home from school, I dropped off at the record department of Lewis's. In those days, presumably when there were a lot fewer records to choose from, the latest LPs would be played aloud in the department for the benefit of all the teens present and the chagrin of any parent who had the misfortune to accompany them. After a few minutes, I was alerted to the song being played because I recognised it as "Blowing in the Wind". But this was different!

The sweetness of Peter, Paul and Mary had been replaced by a background guttral growling, overlaid by words that seemed to be thrown out from the record towards the listener. This was music designed to disturb the consciousness! I wasted no time in establishing, courtesy of information provided by the seventeen-year-old girl with acne behind the counter, that this was Bob Dylan. Not long after my revolutionary insight, Bob Dylan was famous.

I have remained loyal to Bob ever since and have little reason to doubt that the feelings are reciprocated.

Once established in the sixth form, we were expected to behave in a manner that displayed a degree of maturity because things had become a tad more serious. The gesture of recognition of new-found adulthood at that stage was traditionally dropping of the requirement of everyone else to wear a school cap at all times when not in school. Unfortunately, the year that we entered the sixth form saw the rule abandoned for everybody, not just us.

Most of the time we did what was necessary to get the requisite A-levels. We even went into school at weekends to do extra dissection before the biology examination although the effort involved usually had to be compensated by a trip to Tib Lane afterwards - not so much at this stage to the Cona as the Town Hall Tavern next door. The pub was known simply to its friends as the Town Hall.   My father never did understand the connection between a school trip for biology revision and a delayed return caused by a visit to a civic building on the way home.

Perhaps the business of the school caps and the associated failure of the school to recognise our special status caused us to continue to behave in an immature and irresponsible fashion. But regardless it all seemed to work in the end.

It's alright, Ma, I can make it.   Bob Dylan "It's alright, Ma (I'm only bleeding)"

Chapter 2: Germination

The first shoot gives no hint of the nature of the grown plant.

Somehow I got through the Oxford Examination paper and was invited for interview. This in itself was a minor glory because it allowed me to turn a recent failure into somebody else's fault. Stay tuned.

Our new high master at MGS decided that our educational base was not sufficiently broad, which was true as judged by the policy of only taking O-levels of a type and number that would fit us for A-level studies and A-levels that would fit us for Oxford, Cambridge or Somewhere Else but not true when looked at from the perspective of the school orchestra and choral, dramatic and myriad other societies catering for extracurricular interests. Anyway, he decided that all sixth formers should take O-level in general studies, notwithstanding the time constraints generated by the inconvenience of concurrent A-level studies.

I failed, which I guess proved his hypothesis. But here was the catch – the Oxford exam also had a general paper, which presumably I passed. So obviously, the O-level examiners didn't understand what I had written. Any reader who sees a flaw in this argument, please do not write to explain; my tender psyche may not take it.

My turn came and I walked into the interview room where I was confronted by twelve dons sitting in a semicircle. In truth, "confronted" is the wrong word because the door was behind them so that I was greeted by twelve gown-clad backs as my introduction to Oxford academia. One don half turned his head and summoned me into the arena created by the arc of chairs. I waited for the lions.

"Please sit in the chair in the corner." I glanced to my right and saw one chair wedged into the corner of the room and another directly in front of it. Was this a test of intelligence or slavish obedience? Was I to climb over the first chair and sit literally in the chair in the corner or go for the clearly more rational option and sit in the front chair? I opted for the latter. The first phase of my assessment was over but the dons fixed in passive expressions provided no clues as to my success or failure in the task.

I don't remember much of the rest of the interview so I imagine it was boring. Towards the end, the don on the left wing of the team asked me if I had any criticism of the medical profession. My reply that it was perhaps too conservative – "with a small c, that is" – transformed twelve immobile men into a wobbling, shoulder-shaking embodiment of hilarity. I still don't think it was very funny but I am sure it was crucial in getting my scholarship. Perhaps the idea that medicine could be too conservative with a *large* "c" really is hilarious for an Oxford don.

Brasenose College is one of thirty-eight colleges and six halls in Oxford where undergraduates can conduct their academic pursuits with vigour, well for three eight-week terms per year anyway. Actually, for medical students, most of the work is carried out in the science area where students of like discipline from all the colleges congregate each day to pore over a dead body or carry out some other requirement of the preclinical curriculum, that is the period of study before they see real patients.

People ask why doctors only marry doctors or nurses and the answer is that they never meet anyone else. (If you are a doctor reading this and are married to an advertising executive, mole hunter or surf instructor, please do not write to me. I was making what we in the medical profession call a generalisation). There was little chance of finding a spouse in college in 1966, even if your studies were based there, because they were all single-sex colleges and your choice of partner was therefore limited. Even if you were gay, you would not be able to find a spouse because this was long before the period of civil marriages for same-sex couples. Moreover, homosexuality did not become legal until 1967 so, if a gay man went to college in 1966, his first year would have been one of either sex-starved Puritanism or happy criminality.

It comes as a shock on your first arrival at college to be told that you will be spending the next year (apart from the twenty-eight weeks at home) on staircase 11, but the idea of living the life of the homeless with a blanket, dog and a copy of Gray's Anatomy is soon dispelled when you realise that there are rooms off the staircase.

I was a modest, good-humoured boy. It is Oxford that has made me insufferable.   Max Beerbohm

I was told by one of the dons that Brasenose was a middle-class college, by which I assumed that it had only a moderate number of undergraduates from public school. My five friends and I went up to Oxford together from Manchester Grammar School. In those days, the school cultivated (or at least produced) a certain character of student: intelligent, meritocratic, and with a cynical disregard for pretentiousness. That is, apart from those of forms Lower 4th and Lower 5th who were largely ignored. This background equipped us with the ability to cope very well in, and profit from, the Oxford environment because we knew we were at least as good as everyone else (actually better).

Our cynical disregard for pretentiousness was matched or bettered only by that of the college scouts, who were employed to do all manner of things (mostly decent) in the guise of looking after the young gentlemen. For a young Northern lad, of modest upbringing, being woken every morning by a middle-aged gentleman comes as a totally unexpected aspect (I hesitate to say bonus) of undergraduate life.

My scout, Will, was either very clever or very stupid. His morning greeting comprised a statement of the time recorded by my clock, the time recorded by his watch and a conclusion as to how fast or slow was my clock. The slight arrogance in the assumption that his watch was always right was offset by the fact that his calculations of the difference in time between his watch and my clock were universally wrong. I never worked out whether he was so daft as to never get the calculation correct or so smart as to use this as a ploy to stir my consciousness.

It may be a truism for all careers that the most successful people tend not to be the nicest. I don't think Will had any unpleasantness about him but the chief scout was a different kettle of fish. He policed the entry into the dining hall, where we were required to eat twice weekly. All students had to be within the hall by 6:45 or 7:30 p.m., depending upon the sitting, and anyone arriving after that time would be barred from entry. The chief scout's turning away of latecomers was accompanied by a belly laugh through gritted teeth, quivering of the shoulders and conveyance of information that he did not make the rules. His mode of communication was similar for those who failed to follow the rules of attire, which demanded the minimum of a student gown and a tie. Failure to be so clad would deny one dinner, at least in college, a snub marginally less insulting than the mode of its delivery by the chief scout. The rules were strictly enforced to the point of sartorial inelegance; shorts, polo neck sweater, tie and gown were acceptable but a three-piece suit with a gown but no tie was not. I suspect that wearing nothing but a tie and gown would get you into the hall although the police might have something to say about it.

When we did get to eat dinner in hall, it was rather good. At least, the part that reached our plate was; I cannot speak for the portion spilt down our backs by the scouts who served us. I suspect the requirement to wear gowns for dinner was necessitated by this unfortunate habit of the scouts which reflected either an unvoiced contempt for the "gentlemen" whom they served or a remarkable and repetitive clumsiness.

The college hall was the first place (and possibly the only place, come to think of it) that I ate greengages with shortbread as pudding and that alone made me feel as if I had entered a rather elite establishment. The sense of occasion was enhanced by the grace before dinner which was read in Latin by the bible clerk at very high speed, I suspect because he was starving hungry and wanted to get to his dinner. I have never learnt Latin so the grace was incomprehensible and possibly more impressive for that. We could also buy beer in solid silver engraved tankards which, one must admit, is not an everyday experience.

It is generally quite impressive how well students get on together. This is not just because of similar age, intelligence and probably academic pursuit but also a corporate feeling of being part of a separate social group, the "union" or "club" mentality.

We were no exception. We made new friends within college, often those who lived on the same staircase, and in our lectures, tutorials, practical classes and cigarette-smoking and coffee-drinking interludes between them. Jock and I, who went together to Brasenose from MGS, only really took exception to two people who seemed, at the time, the epitome of arrogance, inflated self-importance and swagger. Their favourite sport was to throw bread rolls over the back of the pictures in the dining hall, as they leaned on their hangings at an angle from the wall. I don't know why we objected to this so much because we had not developed a philosophy that specifically forbade damage to paintings or bread rolls. I would like to think it was some form of innate goodness on our part but I may be overstating the case. Anyway, we didn't like it.

We called our two friends Napoleon and Snowball, after the pigs in Orwell's "Animal Farm" that took control. Napoleon and Snowball never really did anything to offend us, apart from the sport of bread and pictures, and even that offence is questionable. We just didn't like them.

I almost gained revenge against Napoleon (why for, for goodness sake?) through his girlfriend, Susan. We did not share Napoleon's friends directly but it transpired that Susan also formed part of a social group of which we were members.

I am now fairly confident that Susan fancied me. She certainly called round to my room on one evening without invitation, ostensibly on her way to see Napoleon (who, of course, also lived in college). I do not know why she lay on the floor at my feet but I suppose I should have suspected something when she started to take her dress off. The problem was that she told me she was showing me how much weight she had lost, not that she could ever have needed to lose any, and I believed her. If I had been Nelson and that had been my Waterloo, history would have been rewritten by my failure to act.

Computers often have a "restore" function so that, if something goes wrong, you can turn the system back to when it was functioning well before the fault wrecked everything. Without being irreverent, I thought I would make a suggestion to God that he missed out on something by failing to install a restore function into the human design. If he had, we would all be able to go back to the fork in the road where we took the wrong turn and choose the right one instead. We would be able to avoid situations that had let us astray and avoid problems before they occurred. If I had a restore function, I would be able to go back to that evening when Susan visited, and grab the opportunity (or, in this specific case, Susan). Fortunately, I have heard other sorry tales from people about experiences in their late teens and concluded that students are not as smart, worldly wise and self-satisfying as they or the rest of the world would like to believe.

Oxford is well known for its high level of academic discipline but, as a medical student, it is easy to forget the intellectualism when immersed in what is essentially a vocational subject. We certainly didn't have the outlook of the young don at an introductory sherry party, who informed us with some self-satisfaction that he was studying number theory. When quizzed whether this was of any practical value either now or in the future (the latter allowing him to claim that he was contributing to the pool of human knowledge), he asserted confidently, and with no shred of concern, that it was not. A further enquiry as to why he was studying something of no practical value led to the reply "Don't you like knowing things?" which brought a riposte from Jock: "Not for its own sake, no!" It's obviously not true for most people but it reflected the medic's attitude to academia, at least in the black and white thinking of an arrogant eighteen-year-old.

There may have been a degree of medical paranoia too. It is easy to confuse intellectualism with abstraction; that is, the more removed a subject is from practical life, the more intellectual it is deemed to be. Medicine does not sound as intellectual as Ancient Greek or philosophy. You use your body to live and your brain to think. Even though many of the famous Oxford scholars were, in fact, physicians, there may have been some such thinking early on in the minds of the organisers of the medical course because, by the time that we entered the University, one could only obtain a degree in medicine if one collected a degree in some other subject along the way. For most people, this was animal physiology, I imagine because it was deemed to be most relevant to clinical medicine. Personally, I would have thought it a better basis for being a vet but never mind. The net result of this requirement was to extend the length of the course from five years in most medical schools to six and a half in Oxford. The extra bit was to allow you to get your preclinical studies up to a level that qualified for degree status in its own right. The University did make up for it though by handing you an MA for no extra work, but at a small price, three years after obtaining your first degree.

Analyzing humor is like dissecting a frog. Few people are interested and the frog dies of it. EB White

Preclinical study essentially involves the workings of the normal body before it goes wrong (which is when you have to know something about medicine). One of the most well-known fields to a lay person is anatomy and, in particular, the special requirement to dissect a human body. Although most bodies were bequeathed to medical research and study, we did not really know that at the time and it added to the considerable mystique of the whole exercise not to find out. Lack of knowledge allows the imagination to run wild and it becomes great fun to speculate by quite which process the body came to be lying in front of you.

The bodies were laid out in slabs and we worked in teams, four to a body. The teams, and the body to which they were allocated, did not change throughout the course. Thus, particular social groups were established serendipitously in the dissection room, one at each body. There would be intermittent comments and questions between the groups, rather like the crews of adjacent ships passing the time of day across the water that separated them. Despite the surreal surroundings, romantic relationships were even established in this way. Indeed, Mike's lasting marriage was spawned by the air of romance spreading between two adjacent dissecting tables.

It is not certain how valuable was the whole dissection exercise, social benefits apart. Specifically, it is very unclear how much it taught us about anatomy. Judging by our knowledge of anatomy at the time of the relevant examinations, the benefit was slight indeed. However, the possibility cannot be excluded that vast swathes of information were embedded into memory by the exercise only to be rapidly eradicated by the fumes of formaldehyde used to preserve the bodies.

In truth, these fumes were quite powerful irritants to the eyes, nose and probably any other delicate membrane with which they made contact. One student resorted to wearing a man's handkerchief tied across her face like a yashmak. Another protected her nostrils with wads of cotton wool so large that they protruded prominently onto the upper lip. A third wore swimming goggles, a not-so-fashion accessory that unfortunately earned her the epithet "Goggles Georgina". I suppose, on reflection, that it could have been formaldehyde that caused one of them later to go mad. Or maybe it was the madness that led her to the alternative dress code. (Who knows?)

Part of the reason why I believe that we learnt very little anatomy from dissection is that it was quite difficult to find and identify what you were looking for. We had a mildly helpful instruction manual. We also had a useless supervisor, usually a postgraduate student making money on the side.

The anatomy of the body which is dead and fixed in formalin is fairly distorted compared with the same structure in life so even familiar anatomical landmarks can look quite different in those situations. This point may not have been grasped by our less-than-helpful supervisor whose sole contribution to helping us find the clitoris was to inform us that we could no doubt find it in the dark. (Even if that were true, it does not necessarily follow that you could find it in the light because touch and vision are quite separate sensory systems, as I learnt in first-year physiology.)

I wonder anybody does anything at Oxford but dream and remember, the place is so beautiful. One almost expects the people to sing instead of speaking. It is all like an opera.
William Butler Yeats

I loved Oxford and most of the time we lived the life of Riley. The High, The Broad, The Turl, Brasenose Lane and South Parks Road were streets that we walked daily. The Trout and The Bear were pubs that we could enjoy without fear of findings ourselves in the Town-and-Gown conflict (some people in Oxford did not like students). St. Giles Fair, Blackwell's Bookshop with its mile length of bookshelves, the college balls, the college buttery, where each afternoon we were served tea, toast and jam, and the immaculately manicured college lawns contributed, in major or minor respects, to the pleasures of being in Oxford. Even the work was fun because everything was a new experience, shared with others of like mind.

College was home, the place to which, as a science student, you would retire after a day's work outside. Tommy was a regular visitor to Brasenose, being a friend of Ian, one of my own close college friends. He exploited the Brasenose delights. On summer afternoons, he was often to be seen lying on his back, with tea to his left and buttered toast to his right, performing pelvic thrusts towards the sky. He was showing the college his action, he once explained.

His other claim to fame was an entrepreneurial instinct rarely found in a philosophy undergraduate, I suspect. Each year, the Freshers' Fair exposes new undergraduates to a vast array of manned stands, tempting them to dedicate their intelligence to great causes, such as one of the armed forces.

In Tommy's second year, the weather was unseasonably hot and the effort involved in constantly having to extricate oneself verbally from one or other of the career vendors led many undergraduates to develop a severe case of what we in the medical profession call thirst. No drinks were on sale so Tommy came to the rescue by buying several crates of lemonade and selling them on to the undergraduates at a fifty percent mark up. He also tried to develop a business marketing a cute line of coiled metal spring bookends. I wonder what became of him. I certainly can't see him as a latter-day Bertrand Russell.

The best balls were the commemoration or "commem" balls, which took place every five years or so and were bigger and better than the rest. All colleges had commem balls but not in the same year, so there was a good chance that you would get to at least two during your undergraduate time in Oxford. There is something special, if not healthy, about walking into breakfast holding a bottle of champagne after a night in the company of Pink Floyd, Creedence Clearwater Revival and Georgie Fame. An ill-fitting nine-pound-sterling dinner jacket from Louis Gross Warehouses and the occasional discarded item of women's underwear in the college grounds completed an air of indulgent decadence.

The truth is that Oxford is simply a very beautiful city in which it is convenient to segregate a certain number of the young of the nation while they are growing up. Evelyn Waugh

Only the exams seemed to put a damper on things.

Oh the exams! Most of the people I knew admired the people we did not know because they seemed to be the ones who worked steadily throughout the course and were fully prepared by the time the exam came round. Others, like ourselves, seemed to leave things inexcusably and impossibly late before starting revision with any seriousness. There is something quite dispiriting about sitting on a bed with a pile of revision notes on one side and a smaller pile of notes that have been read on the other. Ostensibly to plan out my time (but probably in truth, to avoid any work), I started each revision session by calculating how much time I had available for each sheet of revision notes. Unfortunately, having left things too late, there was simply not enough time available so the average time per page decreased progressively as the exam approached, leaving six seconds per page for the final week of revision.

Somehow, something worked because Oxford examiners are not known for their generosity and our crew at least got through. Some employed specialist techniques to gain success. In his anatomy viva, Andy was given a clavicle (collar bone) and told to position it in the orientation that would exist in the normal human body. He told us that he held the bone at its ends, between his two hands, and very slowly rotated it in three dimensions until he was told by the examiner that he had got it right. Knowing Andy, the story was probably completely fabricated and anyway I cannot see how that technique would have helped him in most of the written papers. Turning a pen round and round between the two hands whilst deep in thought may be a common sight in examination rooms but I cannot believe that it helps to produce a good written answer.

In the 1960s, people took acid to make the world weird. Now the world is weird, and people take Prozac to make it normal. Anon

It has been said that if you remember the 1960s, you were not there but we had no experience of drugs, not because we were particularly virtuous or lacking experimentation, but simply because we were not offered any. For most of us, that is. One chap, who lived down the corridor close to my friend's room in Magdalen College was said to be flying high most of the time on LSD but he seemed quite normal to us. Maybe that reflects more on our mental state than demonstrating a reliable and objective assessment of his state of drug intoxication. We were even fairly temperate in alcohol during those preclinical years but we made up for it later in clinical school, where we did everything necessary to prepare for being a doctor.

John, our one-time physiology tutor and a postgraduate student, told us that he had taken amphetamines to keep him awake during revision for finals. The drugs worked brilliantly and he romped through the material into the early hours of the morning but, unfortunately, could remember none of it the following day. Moreover, he felt tired and ill for at least forty-eight hours. Mental note: skip amphetamines in the drug experimentation programme.

I still have a vision of Fifi, sitting at the bottom of a book shelf in the science library, stroking, as she always did, her straight blonde hair with her right hand and never quite making eye contact. Fifi told me that she had been rusticated for smoking cannabis. To clarify, rustication is not a medieval torture or a new experiment in sadomasochistic sexual indulgence but the process of being temporarily "sent down" from the University, usually for a year.

For a moment, I wondered if we now had an explanation for her constant dopey appearance but decided she had probably always been like that. I also preferred that explanation because it showed the manifestation of a rather attractive personality trait and I didn't like the idea that abstinence from drugs would change my vision of her.

She was a pretty girl. She once suggested that we meet when she went up north in the Easter vacation to visit her grandmother. She gave me the telephone number but, by the time I got round to calling, she had gone back home. I didn't follow it up. Don't know why. I missed her in the year that she was away but, by the time she came back, things seemed to have changed.

The establishment of a relationship with Fifi (or anybody else), whether for pure sexual or deeper motives, was not helped by the domestic arrangements that had developed by the third year at Oxford. With the cold but loving calculation of a parent who believes that children succeed best when things are made somewhat but not impossibly difficult, most of the colleges threw out their undergraduate members on to the streets in the third year to fend for themselves. (I am afraid that the true reason is more likely to be that there was insufficient room in college but the argument of social intellectualism is more interesting.)

Fortunately, we had two years' warning of this development and were able to take the steps necessary to put in place the seamless move from college life to the Real World, even within our busy schedules that sometimes included work and without the assistance of our scouts. Four of us found a house to share in Long Hanborough, about eleven miles north-west of Oxford (and two miles from Bladon, whose main claim to fame is that Winston Churchill's grave can be found there). This was a very long way to walk; the bus service was poor; and, unlike the others, I had no car. Quite why I had thought this a good arrangement is now beyond me. I blame my mates. Fortunately, they were good enough friends to give me a lift to and fro - and they had the decency not to jeopardise a medical career by leaving the protege stuck at home like Cinderella. But the lifts did not readily adapt to a love wagon for me and some potential female, especially when they were given by Guy, who had a two-seater Lotus Elan. And the idea of one of my friends bringing the girl to me waiting at home seemed altogether too much like some form of prostitution.

Never mind - by the fourth year, we had decided we were not yet ready for the country life and moved back into town. But, by then, I had hardly seen Fifi for twelve months and her rustication for twelve months had put her into a different year and hence different social group. Nothing ever did develop. Another lost opportunity.

The pangs of your sadness will pass as your senses will rise. Bob Dylan "To Ramona"

Chapter 3: Growth

The most essential part of a student's instruction is obtained...not in the lecture-room, but at the bedside. Nothing seen there is lost; the rhythms of disease are learned by frequent repetition; its unforeseen occurences stamp themselves indelibly in the memory. Oliver Wendell Holmes, M.D.

The student begins with the patient, continues with the patient, and ends his studies with the patient, using books and lectures as tools, as means to an end. Sir William Osler

Growth may mean getting bigger but not necessarily better.

Having mastered the arts of anatomy, physiology and biochemistry (or at least somehow passed the exams), we moved onto the clinical course, which, in contrast to the preclinical course, teaches you about diseases and their treatment, that is what most people would consider as medicine. One might wonder why it is necessary to spend three years learning about how the body functions normally and that would probably be a fair thought. You could argue that you could pick it up along the way whilst doing clinical medicine on the grounds that the normal function is what is *not* going on when disease is present (probably not quite true but it's a good thought).

I believe the modern medical courses do not dwell on these preclinical subjects so much. Moreover, whereas in our day nobody would let you near the door of the medical school without an A-level in chemistry, it is now possible to enter medical school with a degree in media studies. Such is progress.

Most medical students from Oxford went to one of the London teaching hospitals to undertake their clinical course but a significant minority of us remained in Oxford where we were joined by a similar-sized cohort from Cambridge. Although it was rumoured that Cambridge had a university, it certainly did not house a clinical school so the Cambridge preclinical students had to go somewhere and many of them chose Oxford. I cannot remember whether we had anyone from any other universities but, if we did, they were in the distinct minority compared with The Oxbridge Mafia.

The clinical course is really the first time that patients have the dubious honour of being exposed to medical students so the clinical school is usually situated in or near a major hospital. The Oxford Clinical School was based at the Radcliffe Infirmary. Most of the time was spent in the hospital, where not only the patients but also the lecture theatre was situated. However, we did have a bolt hole in the hospital grounds, known as Osler House, which was a quaint old building with several rooms, including a sitting room, toilets and, importantly, bar. There was also a bar-billiards table, bar-football table and a garden where the frustrations of the day could be vented on a croquet ball. Sadly, I never learnt the rules, which may explain my unresolved chronic anxiety state.

The bar was manned by Mr. Haynes. Actually, I believe he was technically the caretaker of Osler House but I don't think he took care of much apart from the bar. He was a skinny man, with slightly thinning, straight, swept back hair and a wizened face and pointed nose. His cheeks were purply red; even though my medical knowledge increased progressively during my time at Osler House, I never worked out whether the facial hue was a reflection of heart disease or chronic alcoholism.

Mr. Haynes was an excitable man. I suspect he suffered from obsessive-compulsive disorder because, if everything did not go exactly according to plan, he became very agitated. Not going according to plan would include a disorderly queue at the bar or two people talking to him at the same time. His reaction consisted of a slight tilting back of the head, half closing of the eyes, downturning of the mouth and the holding of his hands out in front of him ninety degrees from the body. His hands would be afflicted by a rapid up-and-down tremor which made him look as if he was playing an imaginary piano. He looked like a cross between a Dickensian miscreant and a dancing puppet.

All of these idiosyncrasies were well tolerated because he did, in fact, provide quite a good bar service and all on his own initiative. At lunchtime, he brought in sandwiches and fruit pies from Sainsbury's and sold them to the students (probably at a markup). He also fitted out the bar with twelve different draught beers, the taps being positioned equidistant from each other in a line from one end of the bar to the other. These twelve beers formed the basis of the annual "Osler House Run", which involved drinking a quantity of beer from each of the twelve pumps. The winner, who received the celebratory tankard, was the one who could perform this feat in the shortest possible time. There were two competitions: the Major Osler House Run involved one pint from each of the twelve pumps, whilst, for the Minor Osler House Run, the quantity was one half pint. Since the bar was only open from 5:30 p.m. to 8:00 p.m., completing and certainly winning this major annual sports event was quite a feat. This was particularly so considering that the last two pumps in the line were Foster's lager and draught Guinness. The more sensible, or less courageous, of us wimped out.

Apart from the lectures and seminars, and the occasional resort to a book, most of the clinical learning takes place by traipsing around after the doctors, on either working or specialised teaching ward rounds. The difference is that the teaching rounds are devoted entirely to the students, unlike the working rounds where the patients also get a look in. The junior doctors were our everyday partners in crime because they also shared with us the need to progress to the next stage of the career process, which culminated in becoming a consultant.

It is a good thing for a physician to have prematurely grey hair and itching piles. The first makes him appear to know more than he does, and the second gives him an expression of concern which the patient interprets as being on his behalf. A. Benson Cannon

They don't make consultants now like they did then. These people (almost exclusively men) had effectively modelled medical practice through their own efforts, experience and research. Perhaps not surprisingly, the qualities necessary to do that tended to co-exist with other personality traits that include conviviality, good humour, sociability, self-assurance, determination, aggression and ruthlessness (not necessarily in that order of appearance). All of these characteristics seemed to be mixed in with a larger or smaller dash of eccentricity.

Consultants can be broadly divided into two groups according to speciality: surgeons and physicians. Surgeons operate but physicians treat by non-surgical means, usually drugs, conditions such as epilepsy, diabetes, pneumonia and heart failure. There is a (mostly) good-natured rivalry between them. Surgeons believe that they can do everything a physician can do and operate as well. Physicians believe that they do all the important work before and after an operation and surgeons are all right as long as they just cut along the dotted line. It has also been said that the difference between a surgeon and a physician is that a surgeon is someone who has no confidence in nature's powers of healing preoperatively but every confidence postoperatively. The kind interpretation is that this sort of banter stems from territorial instincts and is linked to the qualities necessary to be a consultant.

Rodney Potts was a fairly typical surgeon from those days: his manner was as smooth as high-quality motor oil; his voice was deep and resonating and his complexion permanently tanned and all the more noticeable because of the contrast with his milk-white hair. Someone told us that his permanent tan came from his passion for sailing but, if so, given its permanence, it makes you wonder how he managed to fit in any operations.

Mr. Potts was a vascular surgeon, that is someone who operates on blood vessels. His stock-in-trade was varicose veins, which, together with his appearance and demeanour, made him the lady's darling. The business of the ward round was punctuated by frequent effusive thank-you speeches from his patients, exceeded in frequency and intensity only by an Oscar ceremony.

A senior registrar is a hospital doctor one grade below consultant. Although one might expect that such a person would show blossoming consultant qualities, this was certainly not the case for Mr. Potts' senior registrar, Donald. He had obviously had difficulty getting a consultant post because he looked well past his sell-by date and actually rather older than Mr. Potts who had been a consultant for quite some time. Donald had an ashen complexion, balding head, slightly bent posture and a quiet monotonous voice. Mr. Potts' attitude towards him was of a master to some lowly servant whose dismissal was prevented by some obscure employment law. I suspect that Donald (or Don as Mr. Potts called him) did all the work while Mr. Potts went sailing. By the way, Mr. Potts was always known as Mr. Potts.

Jon Jack, also a surgeon, had a presence that was as difficult to ignore as that of Mr. Potts but he chose quite a different way to express it. Mr. Jack was tall and thin, almost to the point of being gangly. On ward rounds, he made a habit of holding forth to anyone who would listen on subjects that included not only medical matters but also ranged through politics, music, work/life balance and the key defining features of hospital administrators. As he gave these soliloquies, he would adopt a series of demonstrative poses, often leaning with his weight on one leg with the other held at an angle slightly behind him and resting on its toes. His arms would be held out slightly to the side of his body or one arm would rest vertically by his side and the other would adopt a posture as if pointing to the sky. He looked as if he was a crane fly performing Swan Lake. Jon Jack was a general surgeon, that is he undertook most forms of surgery. Indeed, he was wildly opposed to the increasing trend of superspecialisation: "Not much bloody good if you're on board ship, somebody breaks a leg and you say, 'Sorry, I only know about steroids.'"

It seemed as if the physicians were generally quieter and less impulsive although I may have been developing increasing bias.

Samuel Bywater certainly exemplified the distinction from surgeons. He was rotund of both face and body, sported a thick walrus moustache and smoked twenty Benson and Hedges per day. His working hours seemed different from any other consultant. In the morning, he stayed at home and worked in his garden, arriving at the hospital about lunchtime. He fitted in a lot more work than the average consultant (which was considerable) by staying at the hospital late into the day and even night. A particular habit of his was to take a break in the late evening to recharge his thoughts and he would typically go for a walk in the streets around the hospital. On one occasion, he stared upwards in order to gain inspiration but unfortunately was outside the residential block of Somerville College, a ladies' college, at the time.

A helpful policeman arrested him for voyeurism. The claim that he was a consultant physician at the Radcliffe Infirmary was met with a derisive laugh, "Yes and I am the Chief Constable" and accompanied transport to the local police station. His research fellow became his guardian angel by going to the station and confirming his identity. If only Dr. Bywater had altered his appearance to be more like that of the surgeons, and had stopped wearing a grubby mac to walk around town, events may have taken quite a different turn.

Despite his unconventional ways, Samuel had a brilliant mind. His speciality was endocrine diseases, that is diseases of the glands, such as diabetes, and he introduced a number of innovations in both clinical practice and research that set the trend for clinical practice and research that have persisted to this day. He was also a great teacher even though it was necessary to accompany him on his late evening ward rounds to benefit from that quality.

Samuel Bywater's ward rounds were big. On one occasion, I counted twenty-one people following him around the ward or wards (because he tended to have patients scattered across a number of wards). I am not sure where these people came from although some of them were recognisable: registrar, senior house officer, house officer, research fellows and nurses but I don't believe that they accounted for them all. I suppose the rest of them could have been from Rent-A-Crowd to increase the sense of occasion. Anyway, wherever they came from, the net effect was impressive. Samuel would lead from the front, followed by everyone else in decreasing order of importance. Nobody told us where our position should be; it just seemed obvious that, as students, we should be at the back.

Samuel did not spend long at the bedside and preferred to discuss the cases in a seminar room away from the ward. Thus, he walked up to each patient, shook them by the hand, smiled warmly and said, "We are just going to talk about you" before walking off. Inevitably, this meant that the time spent on the ward round itself was short. The brevity of the round and the size of the retinue led to the situation where we, at the back of the queue, were entering the ward just as Samuel was leaving it in the opposite direction. Dutifully, we split into two flanks and Samuel walked between us, followed by the rest, until all we had to do was turn on our heels to take up our position ready for the walk to the next ward. The whole manoeuvre resembled a lesser-known Scottish reel.

The mini-symposium was organised by Samuel as a regular event and designed to train students in public speaking. For our turn, we were given the subject of "Self-poisoning" or, in other words, attempted suicide by drug overdose. This was quite an important subject, in fact, because quite a large proportion of emergency admissions to hospital are cases of self-poisoning.

"There are six of you and I want each of you to talk for ten minutes on a particular aspect of the subject of self-poisoning" explained Samuel. "Your topic, Harvey, will be the acute treatment of self-poisoning."

"But that's a huge topic", I protested, albeit with some relief that I was given a topic that I knew something about. "I could talk for half an hour on that." "Ah, that would be easy" explained Samuel. "But I want you to talk for just ten minutes."

Such wisdom! It is very difficult to tell a coherent story in just ten minutes. I was reminded of that comment on many subsequent occasions when I was preparing talks or presentations at research conferences.

Clinical school – the consultants, the patients, the beer – and, oh yes, the nurses. Being a teaching hospital, the Radcliffe had not only a clinical school but also a nursing school, again situated in the hospital grounds. Every year, a new cohort of eighteen-year-old girls would arrive at the nursing school, where they would spend the next three years, mostly in residence. (By the way, all the nurses in those days, at least in Oxford, were female. This may have been a deliberate selection ploy by the authorities so that they did not have to build a separate residence block for men).

How can anybody hate nurses? Nobody hates nurses. The only time you hate a nurse is when they're giving you an enema. Warren Beatty

There is something stirring about having a residential block of young and not-so-innocent girls just yards away from the clinical school. It seemed to me that, as a breed, nurses were remarkably attractive but I may have been looking through sex-coloured glasses. It certainly seemed easier to have a casual relationship with a nurse than a medical student because the chances were that you would not have to spend the next day working closely with them.

Jackie was a beauty. She had dark penetrating eyes, a pretty smile and thick black hair that made her look like a young Elizabeth Taylor with a pageboy haircut. Her figure was one you could die for (although fortunately, in my case, I did not have to go that far). I had first met her over coffee with the ward sister after a teaching session on a surgical ward, company that was inhibiting to say the least. After two weeks of constant anxiety, uncertain how to approach her without rejection, I saw her in the hospital cafeteria and engineered the route from my table to the coffee machine and back so as to pass her table, where she was sitting alone. So manufactured and tortuous was this route that any observer would either have latched on immediately to my intentions or concluded that I was acutely disorientated. She seemed unruffled at my feigned surprise at bumping into her and happily talked. I guess she knew what was coming but fortunately did not let on and obligingly produced the requisite air of delighted shock at my asking her out.

I had no idea where to take her because I suspected that she knew more about everything useful and fun in life than I did. My friend Ian advised me that it would be cool to take her for a first drink in the Osler House bar before moving on somewhere else because that would show me as a man-about-town or, in this case, a man-about-the-medical-school.

I was too emotionally drained to question the logic of this analysis, which, in retrospect, was almost certainly offered so that he could ogle from the sidelines, and accepted it.

The bar was heaving and desperately uncomfortable, clearly not the place for a first date. After fighting for drinks at the crowded bar, I located a stool for her in the corner by the window and I stood beside her. My pint was downed in a fair instant in an effort to get her out of there as soon as possible. Fortunately, she drained hers equally fast and it was at that point that I learnt that she would always match me drink for drink.

We had a relationship but I am never sure whether we were really going out together or not. We were together on and off for about two years but not continuously. It seemed as if we would be together for a couple of weeks with no plans to continue the relationship subsequently. We would then meet up again by chance, in the hospital, at a party or walking down the street, and resume the same pattern. True, sometimes the lack of forward planning was precipitated by one thunderous row but not always.

She had two defining characteristics: one was to blurt out "Oh my God" every time she laughed. The second was to wear her pants on the outside of her tights. (Americans, please translate "pants (UK)" as "panties (US)" and not "pants (US)" as in "trousers (UK)"; she was English, after all.) I have never met anyone before or since who had this latter facet of behaviour but, for all I know, it may be very common. I am not sure I can quite see the point, though. Maybe it was to cater for the casual upskirt voyeur.

Access to the nurses' block was along a straight corridor from the main hospital, up a flight of about six steps, followed by a one-hundred-and-eighty-degree turn to the left, and then a further climb up another six steps to the first floor. The nurses' rooms flanked the upstairs corridors with an appearance similar to a one-star hotel.

At the entrance to the block on the ground floor, before the first flight of stairs, was an office with a sliding glass door that opened onto the corridor on the left side. This office was manned (or actually womanned) by a ferocious gauleiter who vetted every person who sought to gain access to the nurses' inner sanctuary. You practically had to have a passport to get in and, if you were male, there was little chance unless you could prove that you had come to repair the heating system.

Against this impediment, ingenuity had to prevail. The accepted way of overcoming the hospital equivalent of the Berlin Wall was to start a gentle run down the hospital corridor and accelerate on entering the corridor that led to the nurses' block, so that peak velocity was reached just before the guardian's office. At this point, a well-directed leap would gain a position on the first step of the staircase. Safety was reached on turning the corner in the staircase just a moment later. The technique did incorporate a small gamble that Mother Hen would not be staring straight out through the glass window at the time of the flypast, but, if the moves were executed to perfection, the passing image would have been so transient as to create uncertainty whether she had seen anything or not. Of course, by the time she got out of the office to check, the illegal immigrant had merged into the fabric of the building, specifically one of the nurses' rooms. It was wise only to use this procedure to visit a girlfriend because unsolicited visits would run the risk of police arrest.

Nurses did not remain sweet and attractive as they got older and gained more senior posts (well, not all of them anyway). The sister on Robert Downing ward acted as if she owned the ward and, come to think of it, I have no way of knowing that she didn't. She ruled it with the compassion of a prison guard, at least as far as non-patients were concerned. She particularly hated students. Indeed, we were not allowed onto the ward without asking her specific permission first. If she were absent from the ward when we wanted to visit a patient there, we would have to wait politely in the waiting room until her return. In truth, I don't think she ever left the ward but employed the waiting game as a tactic to exert her dominance. Attempts to enter the ward without her permission were universally pointless because she had such a refined form of student detection apparatus that she could identify our presence within seconds of entering, even if she were engaged in some other task at the time. Rarely would we get more than a few yards down the ward before being halted by a bellowing "Student!" boomed out from the dragon standing, legs apart and arms akimbo, at the end of the ward, with her flushed face jutting forwards from the neck. We did not know her real name but she was known as Sister Robert Downing.

The consultant quirks were on display at the annual Christmas pantomime, where students performed passing imitations of a selection of the hospital's consultants. I was going to say that the students performed a caricature of the senior doctors but they managed to make a fairly good job of caricaturing themselves. The pantomime was called Tingewick, Tyngwyck, Tyngwk or Ptingewick, depending which year it was, because convention had it that the name had to be spelt a different way each year. The show involved a fairly contrived plot around a large pink elephant, called Rita, as a framework on which to make fun of consultants. I never heard of anyone being offended but that may be because the script was vetted by a consultant attached to the Tingewick Society. Editorial strikes were rare although I do recall the excision of "You scratch my back and I'll stick a knife in yours" said from one consultant to another.

The thickly evolving plot was interrupted by songs, written by us, and usually to a Gilbert and Sullivan tune. Piers

Robertson, an obstetrician and gynaecologist, had a notable presence in, or absence from, the hospital:

> *When I was a lad I went to school*
> *And at my books I was no fool.*
> *I got my A-levels 1, 2, 3,*
> *Including a distinction in biology.*
> *I did so well in biology*
> *That now I'm a consultant in maternity.*
>
> *When I was a student I made such a mark*
> *That my chief described me as very best clerk.*
> *I took all the bloods and I wrote up the notes*
> *And I always wore the very whitest of white coats.*
> *Those whitest of white coats did so well for me*
> *That now I'm a consultant in maternity.*
>
> *Now I'm a chief I rarely see*
> *Any patients unless, of course, its privately.*
> *I've made a lot of money and I'll make a lot more yet*
> *But there's one job left in England that I'd like to get.*
> *There's only one job that would really please*
> *And that's to be the man…*

(Set to the tune of "When I Was A Lad" from Gilbert and Sullivan's HMS Pinafore [1878]; new words by Kevin Donnelly.)

The rest of the song is not really suitable for a mainstream book like this but refers to the activities of being the Queen's gynaecologist.

At end of the show, the participants gathered at the end of the hall in various stages of drunkenness to bid farewell to the audience. The manner of saying goodbye varied depending partly upon the degree of intoxication and partly upon the personal preference of the well-wisher. For me, having spent a large part of the previous two and a half hours shaking hands with everyone in sight in bona fide Bywater fashion, it followed naturally to continue the habit with each person at the exit. As my mind began to switch into automatic mode, accompanied by a logarithmic decline in attentional capacity, I took the hand of the next person, smiled abstractly and looked up - into those dark, penetrating eyes that I had come to know, albeit inconstantly, so well.

The rest is cliche, but true. I squeezed Jackie's hand involuntarily; she reciprocated; she said she would indeed come to the after-show party; we danced; and we were back together for a while.

After three years of playing doctor, most of us became real ones and were set loose on the unsuspecting public, rather like a pilot taking his first solo flight in busy airspace. As usual, there was the small hurdle of the examinations to overcome first but very few people failed outright. That does not necessarily mean that everyone who passed ended up being a good doctor.

It is a mathematical fact that fifty percent of all doctors graduate in the bottom half of their class.   Author Unknown

Learning, of course, continues after qualification so the main priority at this stage is to ensure that one is not downright dangerous. In truth, we had also had little choice but to work fairly hard over the previous years.

The education of the doctor which goes on after he has his degree is, after all, the most important part of his education.
John Shaw Billings

Poor Sarah Thompson. She was asked a question about a woman who came into hospital at thirty-six weeks of pregnancy with painless vaginal bleeding. The serious cause of this problem is placenta praevia. In most cases, the placenta, or afterbirth, is attached to the inside of the uterus (womb) some distance from its exit (the cervix) so that it does not get in the way when the baby is born. It placenta praevia, however, the placenta lies close to or, in the worst cases, over the exit from the uterus. As the cervix dilates, the placenta, which is very fragile and full of blood, tends to tear so blood passes out into the vagina. Anything, including a finger, inserted into the vagina at this stage runs the risk of producing torrential bleeding and death of the mother.

"Now Miss Thompson, you are faced with a twenty-five-year-old woman admitted to hospital as an emergency with painless vaginal bleeding at thirty-six weeks of pregnancy. What are you going to do?"

"A vaginal examination, sir."

"That is the one thing you would not do, young lady. Goodbye."

She failed.

I was under the care of a couple of medical students who couldn't diagnose a decapitation.   Jeffrey Bernard

Chapter 4: Nurturing

To encourage growth is to risk producing an unknown quantity.

For those of us who had already decided on a career in hospital medicine, we were about to embark on a long arduous journey of junior hospital posts with no guarantee of achieving the prized consultancy at the end. The progression was from house jobs, through senior house officer, registrar and senior registrar but the process was not guaranteed. Each post had to be applied for and was for a fixed term, after which it was necessary to apply for another post at the same level or hopefully a more senior one. There was no certainty, and in fact only a minority chance, of progressing up this ladder at the same hospital or even in the same city. Thus, a doctor of subconsultant grade would be one of a national tribe of nomads combing the countryside for the necessities of life, in this specific case a job.

The career structure was known as pyramidal which meant that virtually everyone would get their first hospital post, house officer, but thereafter the number of jobs available decreased with increasing seniority. You don't have to be a professional mathematician to work out that this meant that there was a dropout rate that continued right up to the level of consultant. Once that position was achieved, security was assured unless you slept with a patient, raped the matron or said something unpleasant about someone in a position of power. It is no surprise that the gaining of a consultant post led to the popping of many champagne corks.

The first year after qualification was spent in preregistration house jobs, at the end of which doctors achieved full registration with the General Medical Council unless something went horribly wrong. Six months was spent in surgery and six months was general medicine.

I do not know who invented house jobs but I suspect their origin dates back to the time when, in order to be a proper soldier, you had to lose at least one arm. The job was exciting and enthralling but pleasant? No. To be fair, I do not have any specific memories of unpleasantness, more a general impression of constant fatigue.

I was lucky enough to be given both the surgical house job and the medical house job immediately after qualification, with the surgical job to be done first and the medical job second. Unfortunately, the surgical job was in Bath, some sixty miles away, whilst the medical job was in Oxford.

The surgical job involved being on call on a one-in-two rota. This meant that the work programme involved five full days each week, every other evening and night and every other weekend. Being "on call" is a misnomer because it implies that one can sit around except for the rare occasions when someone might need you. In fact, being on call meant not only the requirement to deal with problems that might crop up out of hours within the hospital but also being available for acute admissions. By their very nature, these were emergencies, at least in principle, so each patient would need to be questioned, examined and investigated as soon as possible after arrival, whether by day or night. Many patients would undergo surgery during the evening or night. Sleep was therefore spasmodic and inadequate for a houseman on call. The zenith for this sadistic training programme was every other weekend because the work would extend continuously from Friday morning to Monday evening with very little break.

A few months into my first house job, the Government brought in "extra duty payments" (or overtime) for junior doctors. Payments were allowed (at standard rate) for any time worked in excess of one hundred and eight hours per week. The claim form had to be signed by one's consultant so it was wise to check that their approach to junior staff had advanced at least partially into the twentieth century.

A group of hospital workers that is underappreciated is telephone operators, particularly those who work at night. Not only are they working at unsocial hours but they also have to handle calls from patients and general practitioners, who have no desire to telephone the hospital in the middle of the night, and contact the junior housemen, who have no desire to accept their call. Words such as saint and patience come to mind. They were responsible for alerting staff in the event of a cardiac arrest.

A cardiac arrest is where the heart suddenly stops and urgent attention, within minutes, is required if the patient is not to leave hospital in a box. As junior houseman, I formed part of the team that was called when a cardiac arrest occurred in the hospital. At 3 a.m., the telephone rang in my on-call room and did its best, largely unsuccessfully, to rouse me from sleep. I don't remember picking it up but I must have done.

"Hello, Dr. Sagar, cardiac arrest Ward 4."

"Oh really, when?"

"Now, doctor, now!"

The house jobs constituted a year's steep learning curve with first-time experiences, good and bad, following after each other with uncomfortable rapidity. The first time I put up a drip; the first time I took blood; the first time I did a lumbar puncture; the first time I inserted a chest drain. Actually, some of these were done for the first time as a student, particularly taking bloods, but there didn't seem the same sense of final responsibility then because you were, after all, only a student and could not really be blamed if things went wrong. Not so anymore, because you had been licensed to practice.

At three o' clock in the morning, there simply was not anyone to help out if you were unsuccessful in putting up a drip. Yes, you could telephone the registrar and ask him to get up to bail you out but "not the done thing" represents something of an understatement in these circumstances. In truth, there was always someone to call but the feeling most certainly was that there was not. I held the responsibility for the patient and failure to carry out the investigations or provide the necessary treatment felt not only as if it was my fault entirely but also that I acted as arbitrator at the life-and-death crossroads of each patient, not through arrogance but through fear. Moments of delight and moments of anguish flipped in random order.

John Taylor was admitted as an emergency. The general practitioner informed me that he had had difficulty passing water for the last year or two. When he wanted to pass urine, and tried to do so, he had to wait, with member in hand, for thirty seconds before being able to start. (If you time it, you will find that thirty seconds is quite a long time, particularly if you are standing in a public toilet with Percy in hand pointing at the porcelain and little else happening. Some people may get the wrong idea.) The GP also told us that, when Mr. Taylor did pass urine, it tended to dribble out and he had difficulty stopping the dribbling when he thought he had finished. We knew that these were symptoms of enlargement of the prostate gland, which is wrapped around the exit from the bladder and tends to compress it as it enlarges, thereby impeding normal voiding of urine.

Whilst waiting for a hospital outpatient appointment, six months hence, Mr. Taylor had unfortunately stopped passing urine altogether on the day of admission.

The nurses had already drawn the curtains around the bed. As I opened them, I saw someone with the physical appearance and emotional demeanour of someone late in pregnancy, were it not for the fact that the individual was male. His face was flushed and perspiration trickled from his forehead down his temples. He repeatedly changed position, well as best as he could given that his abdomen was swollen to the size of a football. He was in obvious distress.

I had a sudden thought: can the bladder really enlarge to that size? If so, how come that I have to go to the loo so often and pass such paltry amounts each time? Why not use a bit more of the bladder's potential and go, say, once a day?

Anyway, such thoughts were not terribly helpful, at least to Mr. Taylor, so I explained that we were going to pass a tube up through the penis into the bladder to drain off the urine and that very soon all his discomfort would evaporate. It is amazing how circumstances dictate one's feelings because I imagine that, except for those with specialist sexual interests, the proposal of passing a tube up through the penis would not generate profuse expressions of potential gratitude as it does for someone in the plight of Mr. Taylor. What is even more remarkable is the dramatic relief of symptoms that can be produced by a procedure that takes no more than a few minutes. Mr. Taylor's physical and mental state undertook a one-hundred-and-eighty-degree turn, almost as if a light switch had been flipped. The relief of pain and discomfort that occurs virtually instantaneously as the over-distended bladder is emptied is indeed dramatic. One of the more satisfying experiences in medicine, obviously for the patient but also for the doctor.

Unlike cockroaches. I haven't been to all the hospitals in the country so I do not know if they are all infested with cockroaches but either there is a remarkable coincidence between the hospitals that do have cockroaches and the hospitals in which I have worked or they are following me around. I first learnt to detest them with a vengeance when I was in the sixth form at school, working for zoology A-level. One of the requirements of the practical aspect of the course and hence the examination was dissection of the cockroach. (I expect you have no difficulty in seeing the obvious relevance of this task to a future career in medicine but I do. If it is useful, it must be more related to the working environment of the job than to any skills or knowledge acquired from the inner working of the cockroach body). Our school bred its own cockroaches, which was thoughtful. Even more so, however, was that the school confined their habits and breeding to a cockroach nest in the Biology Department rather than supporting free range cockroaches, allowed to wander at will through the school buildings.

Jimmy Biggs was a quiet, composed man (he was a Quaker) and far too nice to be a zoology master. Not a ruffle of anxiety did he show as he plunged his bare forearm into the cockroach nest, scooped up a handful of the wriggling beetles into the palm of his hand and dropped them into a large glass laboratory beaker. This display of superhuman emotional resilience culminated in a virtuoso performance as he deftly, and with remarkable accuracy, flicked the cockroaches, running up his arm, one at a time into the jar before sealing it with a flat piece of asbestos. So satisfied was he with his performance that his face gave a huge beam. I felt sick.

Cockroaches really put my "all creatures great and small" creed to the test. Terri Guillemets

My second major encounter with the cockroach fraternity was when doing a student vacation job in the kitchen at the local hospital. The cockroaches, which in general are nocturnal and avoid the light, were so brazen that they were running around in the daytime. It was wise to see what the chefs were eating for lunch before selecting your own. There were definitely recipes on certain occasions that were avoided by all the chefs but they were not the same ones every time. I never learnt exactly why but I half suspect that one or more of the cockroaches had found their way into places and utensils where they were even less welcome than on the floor.

The final major encounter was in the hospital where I carried out my surgical house job. From time to time, we would have to go to the pharmacy in order to obtain an emergency supply of drugs for one of the wards. Without exception, turning on the light in the pharmacy precipitated a scurry of three or four six-legged creatures back to the woodwork. I have read that cockroaches stem from the prehistoric era. I wish they would go back there.

My medical house job was back in Oxford. I don't remember cockroaches in the pharmacy there but I do remember looking for them assiduously every time I visited it. It was the morning after one of those nocturnal roach hunts that I went down to the ward to start the daily houseman's routine. These days, blood samples for investigations are usually taken by dedicated venepuncturists, sparing the houseman for even more mundane tasks. It is also usually possible nowadays to obtain the results of investigations by using the ward computer to log into the appropriate department where the investigations are carried out and, if the tests have been done, to obtain the results via the intranet. However, in those days, we did not have such sophistication.

The blood samples had all to be taken by the houseman who, for each test, had to decant the blood into the appropriate bottle, label the bottle with the details of the patient and fill in the appropriate investigation form. If you were lucky, someone would come from the laboratory at scheduled times to collect the samples but, if the test was more urgent, it was necessary for the houseman to take the samples down to the laboratory himself (or herself – care with the potential gender discrimination here!) If there was a ward round on that day, the consultant expected all completed test results to be available so the next task was to chase around the various laboratories, asking if tests had been done and, if so, requesting a copy of the results. Clearly, it was necessary to keep some sort of track on all this activity so details of the tests requested and the results had to be entered into the patient's notes. I don't expect that this mindless activity in the lower ranks is unique to the profession of medicine. In fact, I remember reading the apparently true story of one pupil barrister whose main role for a large part of the day was to stand in his boss's office in such a position as to shield the sunlight from his superior's writing desk.

When all these routine tasks had been completed, the houseman then set to work to "clerk in" the new admissions for that day. These are the patients who are not admitted to the hospital as an emergency but as a planned procedure, either for further investigation or for treatment of a non-urgent condition. Sometimes, they are called "cold" admissions, which is an unfortunate term since a proportion of patients are also fairly cold on discharge, on their way to the cemetery.

My first patient that day was Richard, a twenty-one-year-old, whom I found lying on the bed in a side ward. Richard was a quietly spoken young man with blonde hair and pale skin. He had something of an apprehensive air about him which he disguised by preferring to remain quiet when he could. But when he spoke, his soft voice was accompanied by brief, nervous, side-to-side twitches of his eyes. He was clearly worried.

I took the history from him and carried out a routine physical examination. I asked him what he understood about the reason for his admission. It transpired that he had had a number of very severe nosebleeds, prompting his GP to do some tests, which showed there was a problem with his blood. He had been advised to come into hospital for further tests.

When I later read the outpatient notes, I discovered that he was severely anaemic and there was a shortage of platelets, which are a form of blood cell responsible for effective clotting. The shortage of platelets was very probably responsible for his uncontrolled nosebleeds. By contrast, he had a greatly increased number of white cells, which are responsible for controlling infection, but in conditions where the numbers are markedly increased, they tend not to work properly. Richard was to have more blood tests and examination of his bone marrow, the jelly-like substance on the inside of the large bones, which is responsible for the manufacture of blood cells.

I saw Richard each day, as the further tests were carried out. The initial suspicion from his first set of results was that he had leukaemia but the type he had was thought to be rare at his age, usually affecting younger or older people. Finally, the latest test results were obtained. The diagnosis was confirmed.

Then came the worst part of my doctor's learning curve so far. I had to tell Richard not only that he had leukaemia but also that it was a particularly rampant form and would be very difficult to treat. I had no idea what I would say and so made no plans in advance. I simply let the conversation flow in as gentle a way as I could, trying to ensure that we were engaged in conversation and not that I was issuing a monologue. I remember the occasion vividly but do not remember what I said. I did not know how Richard would react but feared that I would generate a distress that I could not control. In fact, he showed very little reaction. I suspect he already knew in his heart.

That conversation took place on a Friday, by which time Richard had developed a fever from an unknown infection, even though he had been barrier nursed; that is to say nursed in isolation with all procedures in place to minimise the infection risk.

I was not on duty at the weekend. When I returned to the ward on the Monday morning, I learnt that Richard had died.

By the time I returned to Oxford, Jackie had qualified and taken a job in the Radcliffe Infirmary. At the time, I interpreted this as some form of divine design but, some years later realised a far simpler explanation, that she would never leave Oxford unless she had to. (She did change her mind eventually, as many of us with cast-iron convictions often do.) We did not need to choose what sort of relationship we would have because, not only were we working in the same hospital, but also, as fortune would have it, on the same ward. Because she was working long hours and I even longer, nothing much existed outside of medicine and so we practically lived together, albeit mostly on a hospital ward. She always seemed to be the nurse who would call me to see some sick patient or to write up some drugs on the treatment chart; it was always her who assisted when I carried out lumbar punctures or other minor procedures on the ward; it was always her with whom I would collide when I went into the treatment room as someone else was coming out; it was always her working a night shift when I was up all night on call. We were certainly emotionally close and lived a quasi-romantic partnership in our hospital home but feelings were rarely expressed overtly and I cannot remember love being mentioned at all. It was if we had settled into the pattern of relationship of a long-standing married couple with something having been overlooked in between.

The house-job year, which consisted of six months in general surgery and six months in general medicine, confirmed the impressions from my student years that I would prefer a career in hospital medicine to one in surgery. Apart from having a minimal interest in the subject, I was no good at it and disliked surgeons. Admittedly, the last two reasons were related to each other, principally because the consultant surgeon for whom I worked invariably laughed at me if I did something wrong in the operating theatre. At our tender age and bottom-of-the-ladder level of experience, we were not allowed to do anything that could really be called surgery to any self-respecting surgeon but we were allowed to lance boils and were required to assist at operations. The latter largely meant holding a retractor, which was a metal device to hold back bits of the body while the surgeon worked on others, and to cut the silk after he had tied a suture. Occasionally, he would let me undertake more complex tasks, such as tying sutures, but it was there that everything went wrong and confirmed my unsuitability to the speciality of surgery once and for all. Have you ever tried tying a knot in a thin thread of silk wearing rubber gloves? I can assure you that, unless you are destined to be a surgeon, it is impossible. Well, it was for me anyway. I was tested on this rather basic surgical technique on three or four occasions. My consistent failure was followed by an equally consistent outbreak of laughter from my boss that made me wonder for a moment whether he developed a similar level of joy from the misfortunes of his patients. I managed to resist spontaneously stabbing him with a scalpel but could not resist my resolve to do medicine.

The next stage was to progress through the junior hospital posts, senior house officer, registrar and senior registrar, at some point picking up a speciality and hopefully a research degree on the way in order to tick all the necessary check boxes required for appointment to consultant. The first hurdle, however, was to gain Membership of the Royal College of Physicians (MRCP), which required success in two examinations, one theoretical and one practical. The MRCP examination essentially covers all aspects of non-surgical medicine. Usually, hospital doctors do not specialise further until they gain the MRCP. A prerequisite for gaining the necessary experience to pass the examination was to rotate between a number of different specialities.

I successfully applied for a senior house job in Sheffield, which provided three six-month periods of work, in cardiology, general medicine and gastroenterology. I had to move from Oxford to Sheffield, of course, but they granted me single-room accommodation within the hospital for as long as I would like it, which, in the event, was not very.

Jackie and I spent the whole of the three days and nights together before I moved. I cannot remember now why we were not working; I would like to think that we organised it that way but things did not usually work like that between us. The seventy-two hours was the longest time we had spent continuously together and it seems now to have been the best. She saw me off still wearing the party dress she had chosen for the nurses' party the night before, not having had the time to go back to her flat to change, and gave me the three peaches that she had bought for herself so that I would have something to eat on the journey. Nothing more was said. The unspoken understanding seemed to be that we would see each other again sometime and not much would have changed.

I had never been to Sheffield before my interview, which was held in December. I travelled there from my parents' home in Manchester, over the Snake Pass, approaching Sheffield from its north side. Although the M62 did exist, at that time a large proportion of lorry drivers had continued their earlier habit of using the Snake Pass to traverse the Pennines. Since there was nowhere to overtake, my journey from Manchester to Sheffield, which is approximately thirty miles, took about four hours, during most of which time I reflected on how it must have felt to be part of a wild-west wagon train seeking fortune in the West (except that I was travelling east).

The Snake Pass was bathed in swirling fog, which added to the splendour of the occasion. As I descended the mountain on its east side, a sign became gradually visible as swathes of cloud moved across its surface. "City of Sheffield", it said. To say it was a surprise would be a great understatement. Nothing looked less like the approach to a city. We seemed more likely to be in the Middle-of-Nowhere or part of Transylvania.

A few miles further on, the reality of the city hit me head on because we were approaching through the steelworks, which were in such a flourishing state at that time that British Steel was losing an average of four thousand pounds per employee per year. There was certainly a lot of activity but it looked thoroughly unpleasant. The provision of entertainment by Sheffield City Council for visitors approaching from the North consisted largely of black smoke, bursts of flame and heavy machinery noise. One wondered where the people lived. It was only after having been in Sheffield for six months, when I ventured out of the hospital accommodation, that I realised that anybody of sufficient wealth lived in the South or West. Until that discovery, which was actually quite pleasant, I had fully understood the claims of the local residents that Sheffield is such a marvellous city because it is so easy to get out of.

Apart from the steel works, my initial impressions of Sheffield may have been influenced by race memories from the Wars of the Roses, having moved from the fiefdom of my birth in the House of Lancaster to work in the House of York. I must have changed my allegiance to the white rose at some point because I stayed in Sheffield to do my research degree and returned after a break as registrar and senior registrar to take up a consultancy in the steel town. I also stopped going to Blackpool, although there may be other reasons for that. I am surprised that I was not tried as a traitor because memories in those parts die hard.

Yorkshire people are the salt of the earth. They are genuine, on the whole honest, straightforward (sometimes very) and have a good sense of humour. Unfortunately, most of the consultants who work in that area do not originate from it and often do not share these qualities. The three consultants for whom I worked as a senior house officer were, however, "of good character", possibly because two came from Yorkshire originally and the other one was Scottish.

Ken Peacock was a wiry, balding man with a retained Yorkshire accent. He loved cardiology. He did not have the traditional air of a consultant, more of a teenage stamp collector whose exuberance at identifying a new stamp is understood by very few other people. Cardiology, perhaps not surprisingly, involves listening to hearts. Ken had raised the skill to its own art form and indeed was very good at detecting heart murmurs that nobody else could hear. Well, that is what he said anyway. We would stand round the bed, armed with stethoscopes, ready to attack the poor patient's chest. I took my turn.

"Diastolic component?" said Ken when I had finished.

"I can't hear it, I'm afraid", I replied.

The registrar took his turn. "Diastolic component?" said Ken.

"I don't think so", said the registrar.

"Aye, it's there." Ken terminated the discussion.

It is surprising, how, if you spend most of the day listening to heart sounds, they can become something of an obsession. I expect a similar experience is shared by a group of twitchers standing in a forest glade trying to identify some distant bird song. Since the bird is rarely seen, there is little way of proving whose opinion on the matter is correct.

Listening to heart sounds was certainly an experience I gained in that SHO job. I did an outpatient clinic with Ken. He would see the new patients and I would see the follow-up patients. Since virtually all the patients under follow-up were there because they had faulty heart valves, usually caused by rheumatic fever in childhood, an essential part of the follow-up was to listen to the heart to determine whether the murmurs had changed or new ones had been created. In truth, since most of these patients came every six months, any one SHO would rarely have seen any of the patients previously. It is difficult to describe a murmur in the clinical notes with sufficient specificity for someone else later to compare their findings with the previous ones, so the whole follow-up exercise, at least as far as listening to the heart was concerned, was of dubious value. Of course, there were other reasons for follow-up, such as to detect any changes in heart rhythm or the presence of heart failure, but listening to heart sounds seemed to occupy the major part of the clinical exercise. Allowing for two weeks of holiday during the six-month period, I estimate that I listened to thirty hearts per week for twenty-two weeks in that clinic alone, which amounts to six hundred and sixty hearts in total. Maybe you can understand why it made such an impression on me.

Ken had a way with words. On a Wednesday morning ward round, about half way through the job, we approached the bedside of John Townley who had been admitted for further investigation because he became easily breathless on exertion. I presented the history and the findings on examination (because it was a specialist area, there was no houseman so I was still bottom of the pile). Ken went through his usual routine of listening to the heart and identifying murmurs that nobody else could hear and glanced at the ECG rapidly as he passed it through his fingers. Picking up the chest X-ray, he moved closer to the bedside so that he could hold the X-ray against the light. By now, he was about eighteen inches from the patient. Ken took a sharp intake of breath after glancing at the X-ray.

"Oh what a terrible heart", he exclaimed, almost gleefully. "Three valves!"

Judging by Mr. Townley's reaction, I am surprised we didn't have to call the cardiac resuscitation team there and then.

The longer one spends dealing with acute or dangerous situations, the more the initial fear and anxiety subsides. "You never get used to it" certainly doesn't apply to medicine. With sufficient experience, a real emergency, where urgent action is required, produces no more tension than dealing with a routine matter in an outpatient clinic. The important thing is to decide what to do and to do it within the time you have available, which is not necessarily as quickly as possible. Until there is realisation of this difference, the demeanour of an experienced consultant in dealing with an emergency can appear as benign indifference.

One of the routine weekly sessions in the Cardiology Unit was cardiac catheterisation, which was an investigation of the state of the heart valves or of the arteries that supply the muscles of the heart. The procedure involved passing a catheter, a small tube, up one of the blood vessels in the arm or leg until it reached the heart. X-ray dye was then injected into the chambers of the heart. Valve leakage could be detected by visible escape of this dye from the heart chambers through valves that should have completely closed to prevent it. Passage of a tube into the heart perhaps understandably irritates the heart and can cause it to beat in abnormal rhythms. The more the heart is irritated, the more abnormal these rhythms become and the more likely is the heart to stop altogether. Thus, a cardiology technician was on hand to monitor the heart rhythm during the catheterisation procedure. She would call out the nature of any rhythm abnormality that was produced. Withdrawal of the catheter back from the heart virtually always abolished the abnormal rhythms. The test of steeliness of the nerves of the doctor was at which point in the development of a series of increasingly abnormal rhythms he would decide to withdraw. Extrasystoles, isolated extra beats, would develop into runs of extrasystoles, a number of extra beats in sequence. More heart irritation then produced ventricular tachycardia, which was a sign of very unstable heart function, to be followed only by ventricular fibrillation, which was loss of any organised electrical activity of the heart, resulting effectively in cardiac standstill.

Ken was the master of the cliffhanger. Without flinching, whilst we were getting more and more hot under the collar, he would continue his investigation as the technician, with equal calmness of voice, spoke:

"Extras."

"Extras running."

"VT."

"VF."

Usually, Ken would stop at VT but I did see him allow progression to ventricular fibrillation before calmly moving everyone from the table and restoring electrical rhythm by electrical shock to the patient's chest, using the cardiac defibrillator which was kept by the side in the event of such an emergency. Normal heart rhythm restored, Ken then continued his investigation without a flinch of expression at any stage that anything untoward had happened. At first I thought this behaviour was foolhardy but I learnt that medicine is essentially a hazardous business, both in investigation and in treatment, so the only way to gain maximum benefit is to know precisely how far one can go to improve matters without making the patient worse. Waiting for ventricular fibrillation may be going a bit over the top, though.

The responsibility given to junior doctors in those days was far greater than it is now, an experience that was at once both exhilarating and downright frightening. It is surprising that there were not more catastrophes; perhaps there were but nobody noticed.

I was not long into the cardiology job before I was carrying out cardiac catheterisations myself. On the whole, things went remarkably well until one day. In order to access the vein to insert the catheter, it was necessary to perform a "cut down" which means making a small incision in the skin so that the vein can be seen. A small nick is then made in the vein and the catheter is inserted through the hole. On this particular day, all seemed to go well. We were investigating the right side of the heart, which, on the whole, generated less in the way of abnormal heart rhythms than left heart catheterisation. As the catheter entered the heart, I heard the technician's words, familiar in another context, "Extras, extras running."

I withdrew the catheter from the heart and, when the rhythm had settled back to normal, tried again. The heart behaved rather better this time so I injected some X-ray dye. The catheter was clearly in the left ventricle and not on the right side of the heart. I stopped the procedure, sifted mentally through my not-so-encyclopaedic cardiological knowledge and concluded that the patient had a hole in the heart so the catheter had passed through the hole from the right side to the left. My excitement at this discovery was dissipated after Ken arrived and informed me that I had inserted the catheter into an artery and not a vein; arteries are connected to the left side of the heart. Ken was left to suture the hole in the artery because, unlike veins, the pressure in the artery is too high for the hole to close on its own. The patient had a good pulse in that artery afterwards and suffered no ill effects. Ken recovered from his initial reaction of anxiety bathed in an air of criticism. I felt reassured at my decision not to become a surgeon.

Nothing I have experienced since has led me to believe that that decision was wrong. Indeed, appropriate events have taken place at sufficient regularity to lead to the conclusion that I was undoubtedly right. When I bought my first car, I decided that I would service it myself, in respect to all the friends of my father (but not my father himself) who serviced their own cars with apparently as much ease as any other routine day-to-day activity. In fact, I think I did it all right but, by the time I had finished, the car was ready for another service. I never tried again. That and a number of similar happenings led me to believe that I did not have a lot of practical ability at all. I could manage painting and decorating but that was about it. Later on, after harbouring years of feelings of inadequacy in this area, one of my mentors told me that he did what he was good at in order to earn the money to pay somebody else to do what they were good at. Pretty good maxim, I thought.

As a junior doctor, you learn not only about the subject of medicine but also about the people with whom you work, other doctors, nurses, secretaries and patients. This is, of course, typical of all jobs that work closely with people but the added feature of dealing with health and disease, and the precariousness of life, seems to make that involvement with the personalities of people more necessary and possibly deeper. This is not always a good thing. I have met a number of people with whom I'd rather not have a superficial relationship, let alone a deep one. In my naivety, I once asked another of my mentors why some consultant had behaved in a particularly obnoxious manner. "Harvey, there is a lot of psychopathy in medicine" was the reply.

My time in the SHO jobs seemed to go remarkably quickly, possibly because eighteen months isn't very long to gain experience in three specialist subjects. The general medicine and gastroenterology jobs I remember as a year of gradually mounting tension, culminating in the MRCP examination. Fortunately, the serious business was punctuated by moments of levity. Philip Parkin, my consultant on the general medicine job, spent the first hour of every ward round sitting in the sister's office, drinking coffee and recounting stories, mostly of his army life, to his junior staff. He certainly had a natural comic wit which was arguably superior to his skills in medicine. He had a great sense of the absurd. He conveyed effortlessly the pointlessness of the army initiation rite in which the young recruit is catapulted by four men down a polished dining table to crash head first into the fireplace at the end. He was not a typical consultant. Apart from his profuse curly black hair, corduroy trousers and Gipsy-like appearance, his beaten up, dirty Citroen 2CV would not have warmed him to most of the patients in private practice, for example.

I cannot tell you much about Donny McClaren, the gastroenterology consultant, because he was not often there. He turned up for the ward rounds but his response to the history and other information conveyed to him by his junior staff was usually a rich Scottish "Aye" or, if he was really excited, "Ooh aye". He was in the last three years of the job before retirement, at which point he would receive a pension that was dependent upon his total earnings in the final three years of his job. He did not supplement his NHS salary with any private practice but had regularly carried out domiciliary visits, which are examinations of patients in their home, at the request of the general practitioner. Such a visit earns a fee. Donny had grasped the nettle with a view to his pension income by carrying out as many domiciliary visits as he could manage in the last three years of his career so he was rarely in the hospital.

He was so successful in this venture that I suspect he placed one of those workmen's advertisement boards outside each house he visited-

> Donny McLaren
> Domiciliaries 'R' Us
> Call for free quote

I decided as a student to specialise in paediatrics but, after qualification in 1972, the higher authorities had decided for some reason that it would be useful for doctors specialising in disorders of children to have expertise in disorders of adults as well. Thus, budding paediatricians had to gain higher qualification in adult medicine before being let loose on children.

The big hurdle for the embryo physician after the medical degree is the examination to gain Membership of the Royal College of Physicians (MRCP). Surgeons have their equivalent Fellowship of the Royal College of Surgeons. Until relatively recently, doctors in all specialities had to belong to one or the other college in order to gain specialist status but increasingly specialities other than general medicine and general surgery have wanted to break away and set up their own empire elsewhere. This is not necessarily a bad thing because, after all, if the Pilgrim Fathers had not had a similar spirit of seeking independence from the Motherland, we would not have the United States of America, with all its virtues, such as Disneyland.

It is not entirely clear why equivalent levels of postgraduate skill and experience are recognised as Membership of the Royal College of Physicians (RCP) but the superior-sounding Fellowship of the Royal College of Surgeons. The RCP does have a Fellowship grade but that is granted years later at the discretion of the College. Maybe surgeons feel that their postgraduate qualification is fundamentally more important than that of the physicians and demands a more meritorious title. Maybe physicians feel that they are capable of ongoing skill development throughout their career, unlike the surgeons; hence, a more senior title is available to recognise this progress. Sadly, the truth is probably nowhere near as exciting and the reason for the difference lies somewhere in history.

The RCP was founded in 1518 when the King was petitioned by a group of physicians led by Thomas Linacre. Its purpose was to grant licences to practice medicine and oust bad practice. The first college was sited at Amen Corner near

St. Paul's Cathedral, an address which hopefully did not reflect on the destiny of patients treated by the College membership. The founding charter stated that the College aimed to "curb the audacity of those wicked men who shall profess medicine more for the sake of their avarice than from the assurance of any good conscience, whereby many inconveniences may ensue to the rude and credulous populace". The College refused to admit candidates from non-Oxbridge universities until 1835 despite an approximately seventy-year battle on the subject. Women were excluded until 1909 but further delays ensued and the first female fellowship was granted in 1934. Not much really changes in medicine.

In the sixteenth century, surgeons were linked up with barbers in the Worshipful Company of Barber Surgeons. Barbers not only attended to the hair and shaving but were also involved in surgical, medical and dental treatments, especially after the Pope decreed in 1163 that members of religious orders should not be involved in the shedding of blood, a practice that was widespread at the time for the treatment of a variety of medical conditions. Surgeons did not have a medical degree or indeed any formal qualification, unlike physicians who had a university medical degree. The surgeons broke away from the barbers in 1745 and, in 1800, a royal charter was given to found the Royal College of

Surgeons in London followed by the Royal College of Surgeons of England in 1843.

The Royal College of Physicians insisted that candidates for the surgical college must have a medical degree first. Thus would-be surgeons had to qualify in medicine and received the title "Doctor". Rumour has it that, once they gained Fellowship of the Royal College of Surgeons, they reverted to their old title "Mister" so as to snub the physicians' college. The tradition of change of title on gaining Fellowship has continued to the present day although the reason has been glossed over in history. The Company of Surgeons that was founded when they broke away from the barbers in 1745 had its premises close to the Old Bailey and Newgate Prison but hopefully this was not designed for the convenience of the fellows travelling between the two.

Physicians diagnose and treat. Surgeons cut and used to be barbers.

The MRCP examination used to be in two parts. The first was a multiple-choice written paper but the second was a clinical examination involving real patients. The two parts were really separate examinations because part two could only be taken after a pass at part one and the two sections were usually taken about twelve months apart.

The only memorable thing about part one is the marking system. One point was given for a correct answer, zero for no answer and minus one for a wrong answer.

Whoever dreamed up that scheme is a virtuoso in sadism because the anguish involved in trying to find the correct answer is bolstered by an undercurrent of anxiety as to how confident one is about it. If unsure of an answer, do you leave it out and get zero or risk being given minus one which effectively wipes out a previous correct answer confidently produced? If the pass mark is fifty percent, the marking system allows a score of seventy-four percent correct and twenty-six percent incorrect, with no omitted questions, to fail but fifty-one percent correct and forty-nine percent unanswered to pass. The system might have had some merit if the questions were all life-or-death type but they weren't. But, you know, if you want to belong to a club you have to play by the rules.

And though the rules of the road have been lodged, it's only people's games that you got to dodge; and it's alright, Ma, I can make it. Bob Dylan "It's alright, Ma (I'm only bleeding)"

Part two of the MRCP examination consisted of a clinical part and a viva. The clinical section had two components – long cases and short cases. These terms did not refer to the size of the box that would carry off the patient in the event of a less-than-ideal treatment plan but to the length of the clinical assessment. We were allowed about an hour on our own with the patient to take a history and carry out an examination, after which we would present our findings to the examiners and await interrogation and destruction. In the short cases, we were taken to a number of patients, one at a time, and were required to examine a particular bit of their anatomy in full view of the examiners, to say what we had found and await interrogation and destruction.

The clinical exams take place at a number of hospitals throughout the country, depending upon whether some keen consultant or other has offered their services to provide an examination facility where they work. The set-up requires no fancy apparatus, just a ward, usual doctors' tools such as a stethoscope and, most importantly, a supply of patients with a variety of conditions each characterised by some key physical signs for the candidate to detect. The patient must be willing to attend on the examination day. The organisation involved, with its necessary advance planning, usually meant that the patients in the exam were not plucked at the last minute from the Intensive Care Unit, breathing their last, but travelled from home where they lived with a stable but probably largely incurable medical condition, blessed with good physical signs.

Many of these patients came up willingly year after year, for largely philanthropic reasons because they received no reward for their services, unless you count the beaming smile of their consultant as some form of recompense. Contrast this situation with that of volunteers for trials of very new drugs. In the first phase (but not later), people are paid for taking a drug previously tested only in animals. The participants are usually required to live at the testing centre for anything up to one month, to take the drugs and undergo regular tests, especially of toxicity. Not many people can accommodate this schedule easily into their life for fear of conflict with their employer, spouse, child or cat but the homeless tend to welcome a few bucks and nights in a warm hospital bed. The inconvenience of taking a potentially lethal drug is apparently worthwhile.

One wonders whether the medical background of the homeless volunteers, which in truth tends to include greater-than-average quantities of alcohol and drugs, is representative of the population who will later be given the treatment. One might wonder further whether the conclusions drawn from these studies can be extrapolated to the general population but we are assured by the pharmaceutical companies that everything is just dandy. Anyway, lots of other people get to test the drug at a later date so there is plenty of opportunity to poison all kinds of different people. Actually, the truth is that these trials, at least in the later phases, are so rigorous that one sometimes wonders how suitable volunteers, who are not excluded for some minor coincidental condition or treatment, can be found. This rigor is one reason why it takes so long between discovery of a new drug and its appearance on the market, available to doctors to prescribe. Another reason is bureaucracy.

Anyway, back to the MRCP examinations, which did not have these restrictions.

I was allocated to a hospital in Croydon, Surrey for my examination. Living in Sheffield, I thought the choice of venue to be what we in the medical profession call inconvenient but I didn't say so. My reasons for thinking so, however, were that the route to Croydon involved a train journey from Sheffield to St. Pancreas Station, London, an underground trip along Victoria Line to Victoria Station, a further railway trip from there to East Croydon Station, a twenty-minute bus trip and a walk, features that arguably satisfy well most definitions of inconvenience.

Arriving early, I found a female soulmate who seemed to be the only other MRCP candidate at that hospital that day. I think she had travelled from Aberdeen or possibly somewhere more distant. We sat on a grassy bank in the blazing sun in conversation for what seemed to be hours until the examiners or their minions called us for a grilling. We were certainly together alone for long enough to have satisfied all the requirements for a chat-up session but we had too much on our minds to follow it through. Anyway, a relationship exercised between Sheffield and somewhere even further north seemed impractical. I wondered whether the examiners plan all this sort of thing in advance to prevent amorous associations developing out of their serious professional endeavours.

Real love stories never have endings. Richard Bach

I was introduced to my long case, Mrs. Hetherington, a pleasant woman of about forty years who was so relaxed and confident that I assumed she had either done this a million times before or was an actress. (Incidentally, these days, the "patients" *are* often actors and actresses but were not then.) I concluded, after some enquiry, that she had had a brain haemorrhage many years previously.   A sense of self-satisfaction on my part induced a state of calm almost to match hers. I went on to conclude my history taking with the routine questions that included details of her past medical history.

"Have you ever been in a hospital for anything else?" I asked.

"I have been a number of times for tests on one of my eyes", she replied in a tone of deliberate mystery.   Sensing atmosphere, I felt an impulse to enquire more deeply.

"What was wrong with you?"

"Nothing really but they saw something that they felt needed investigation."

"Did they see it through one of these?" I asked, showing her an ophthalmoscope, which is routinely used to examine the inside of the eye.

She smiled and said simply "Yes."

"Do you mind if I have a look?"

With her agreement, I shone the light into her right eye and examined the retina at the back of the eye. I saw nothing amiss. I leant slightly over to the left and whispered in her right ear, "Which eye was it?"

"The left," she said with a low, ponderous voice that led me to conclude that she was enjoying a small conspiracy at the expense of the examiners.

As I began to examine the left eye, she moved it into a position that she had evidently learnt best demonstrated the abnormality to an observer such as me because at once I saw, right in the centre of my view, a tangle of abnormal blood vessels, known as an angioma. Then it clicked. Because these vessels are not normal, they are fragile and tend to bleed easily. A similar one inside the brain could have explained her earlier brain haemorrhage.

The examiner seemed satisfied when I offered the diagnosis, albeit tentatively, of Von Hippel-Lindau syndrome, a rare congenital condition characterised by the presence of multiple angioma-like cysts in different parts of the body. It is amazing what reading does for education because it is only in books that I had come across the condition before or, for that matter, since. It is also amazing what diagnoses MRCP examiners thought would be a good testing ground for practical medical skills. I assume it must be more exciting to examine on a condition that not many people are likely to come across ever again than acid indigestion or catarrh, which are common but boring.

The prowess of Mrs. Hetherington and me in the long case seemed to make the examiners positively sympathetic in the short cases. As I gave a half-baked account of the heart condition responsible for the murmur I had detected in a twelve-year-old boy, one of the examiners stopped me abruptly.

"Dr. Sagar, how would you describe the colour of the patient?"

Remembering that this was a clinical examination, I refrained from commenting on the racial origin of the person under discussion and replied, "Blue, cyanosed."

"Exactly," he said triumphantly. "And what does that tell you about a possible shunt in this young man's heart?"

"It's going from the right side of the heart to the left."

"Exactly!" he said with a shade more triumph. "Now can you tell me the origin of the murmur?"

We established together that our young man had congenital heart disease and again together worked out how it was producing noises heard through the stethoscope.

I have never found out whether it has any statistical basis but it used to be rumoured that pass or failure in the short cases was closely related to the number of patients seen. Less than three led to a fail and five or more would be a sure pass. It reminded me of my history teacher at school who marked the essays according to the number of pages written, leading most of the class to copy large chunks from the textbooks, confident of thereby getting a high mark. Anyway, I saw four cases.

The viva was taken at the College premises. My first interrogator informed me proudly that he was a cardiologist (I resisted the temptation to applaud) and so he was going to ask me about cardiology. I could not fault his logic. The second interrogator asked me about diabetic retinopathy, a problem in the eyes caused by diabetes. With some relief at the topic presented to me, I expounded at length all my hard-learnt knowledge about the condition. I sighed and smiled as I finished.

"That's obviously not your favourite subject" he said. "Let's move onto something else."

One could wonder if professional examinations test the ability to withstand psychological abuse as much as anything else but, despite all that, I passed. Thank goodness – although, in the event of failure, there is always the opportunity to go through the whole unpleasant process once more. As one of my mentors put it, "There is no profit from passing the examination first time but every profit in having passed it at all." An afterthought: presumably the psychological robustness of those who, despite repeated failure, take the examination three or four times without giving up is statistically greater than those who pass it first time. Somebody should do the research.

I thought I had pretty much set up my career path in paediatrics from an early stage. All medical students had an elective period of eight weeks during which they could devote their energies to anything of their choice, provided that it was related to medicine. This association was fairly loosely interpreted by most people, the sometimes ingenious medical links allowing them to fly off to the furthest corners of the globe.

"A study of the incidence of tendonitis in Californian surfers."

"Factors influencing the spread of sexually transmitted disease amongst first-year female Italian students."

"Medical hazards of off-piste skiing in the French Alps."

"Is a specific disease profile associated with work in a French vineyard?"

The possibilities were endless. For some reason, I had missed this loophole in the rules when I chose my project and ended up with four weeks in Manchester and four weeks in Oxford, studying the post-mortem reports of over three hundred stillborn children. The pathology departments in which the records were held were unnaturally dark, possibly in deference to the dead. However, as a result, I spent every day poring over records locked away in the dusty archives, sitting at a desk in a dingy corner illuminated by an anglepoise lamp.

As I pondered my misfortune that I had not chosen any more cosmopolitan topic for my elective (how about, "The medical risk of intercontinental air travel"?), I was reminded of my week-long field trip to the Isle of Man when studying biology in the sixth form at school. We all had a project to do there as well. I don't know how it happened but my topic was osmoregulation in crabs. The purpose of this project was to investigate how crabs manage to live in both sea water and the relatively fresher water that can be found further up the shore. You are right, it was not desperately interesting but even less interesting was the fact that the project involved weighing the crabs every five minutes, a commitment that tended to impair one's ability to leave the laboratory. The social mixing between my friends and the girls from Southport High School, who were at the field base at the same time, largely took place immediately outside the window where I was working. The positive influence on adolescent girls of a blatantly sex-hungry young male waving ominously and without subtlety through a window, over a beaker of crabs, is mimimal. At least they had their fun and I had my crabs – and maybe, if they were not careful, they would get their own crabs too.

As it turned out, my medical student elective was a career winner. The research turned out some interesting results which, in 1973, were published in the British Journal of

Obstetrics and Gynaecology. Having the paper published in a mainstream medical journal is unusual for a student and probably helped me get the SHO job in Sheffield. During that time, I also met the Professor of Paediatrics in Manchester, who seemed to take a liking to me and took me under his wing. He formulated the ultimate plan: I would return for an SHO in paediatrics at the University of Manchester, then work with his friend and colleague in Oxford at its famous paediatric research centre. After that, my career would be made. Not a bad idea.

This eminent plan was undermined by a neurologist. As part of the preparation for MRCP, a group of junior doctors, including myself, went regularly to a nearby ward to see neurological cases under the care of a particular consultant, Tommy Shaw. Tommy was technically a general physician with an interest in neurology. That meant that, whilst the majority of his patients had neurological disorders, he also dealt with non-neurological conditions. In fact, if Tommy did have an interest in neurology, it was not clear that neurology had an interest in him. Maybe it depends on how you define "majority of patients". Certainly, at any one time, most of the patients on his ward were neurological but that was largely because they all had strokes and Tommy believed in rehabilitation not so much as a tool to aid recovery but akin to some sort of magic wand that, if kept waving for long enough, would one day lead to a miraculous overnight cure.

Well, he certainly kept the patients on the ward for physiotherapy and occupational therapy long after the physiotherapists and occupational therapists themselves believed they had any more to offer. If we measure neurological interest by the proportion of new patients who have neurological conditions, Tommy would probably have had less neurological experience than his registrar, especially since he didn't see the patients until the ward round, when all assessments and tests had been carried out. But he was a kindly fellow.

To be fair to Tommy, he knew full well the nature of the patients with whom he was dealing and he had no pretensions. On one of the rare occasions when he spoke to us, he told us that it was not his idea to be called a "consultant with an interest in neurology" and that it would probably be more appropriate to be called a "consultant with an interest in everything else". He also suggested that we sit in on "real" neurology clinics as part of our training for the MRCP examination. Thus, once weekly, I made my way down to the Outpatient Department and sat in with Richard Peters. Richard enthused about neurology and conveyed its interest as if there were no other subject worth studying. Having got to know him well later, I think that is truly what he believed. Anyway, he converted me and the rest of my career was set. My carefully constructed infrastructure for a glittering career in paediatrics was blown apart and a neurological monolith had now to be built in its ashes. So back to Oxford.

Chapter 5: Blossoming

Blossoms are attractive fronts for the mundane.

Wednesday mornings at the Radcliffe Infirmary were spent for me in Neurology Outpatients. The clinic started at nine and first on the list was Myrtle Musgrove. This was potentially bad news because I had been in my registrar's post long enough to have seen Myrtle on several of her regular three-monthly visits. Having her first on the list threatened to destroy the whole of the clinic because we had follow-up patients booked every fifteen minutes and she wouldn't get out of bed for a consultation of less than thirty minutes, whatever problem she had. I don't know why none of my predecessors had discharged her from the clinic because it had become fairly clear to me after just a few visits that, although her condition was not perfect, it was unlikely that we were going to be able to do anything further to help her, for a variety of reasons.

Myrtle Musgrove had epilepsy. She was quite unusual because the condition had begun in her sixties and investigation had not shown any reason for the epilepsy, as is often the case in older people but much less with epilepsy of young onset. The unfortunate fact that all the investigations, including brain scans, were normal, did little to assuage her belief that "something was going wrong in her head". Indeed, it was and I tried to explain that the seizures were arising at a microscopical level, similar to an electrical short circuit, which need not show on tests such as brain scans. Unfortunately, this admission of a brain abnormality accompanied by normal test results became magnified and extended to the notion that she had a nasty brain tumour which did not show on the scan, a point of view that she argued with considerable ferocity against any view to the contrary.

She always came with her husband whose anxiety levels exceeded even hers. In fact, she denied having any emotional reaction to her condition at all; "I am quite a strong woman really" she would repeat at each visit, with the characteristic posture of raised eyebrows, closed eyes and head tilted to the left and upwards, her greying black ponytail drooping over her right shoulder. She was a slight woman with a gaunt face, pointed nose and pursed lips. She rarely smiled and, when she did, somehow managed to convey the impression that you should feel guilty at having provoked such an unwanted reaction.

He, by contrast, was tall and large, but not fat, with a round ruddy complexion and an expression that switched randomly from frowning concern to bright-eyed laughter. The concerned expression was universally the one that began the consultation as his wife walked regally through the consulting room door and he followed behind, clutching a sheaf of papers, that recorded in detail every attack that she had had since her last visit.

"We have had some more doctor", he said woefully, shaking his head. "I wonder if we should change her treatment." This suggestion occurred at every consultation and I was never sure whether his opinion on the matter was shared by her. She certainly never gave any indication. In fact, she spent most of the consultation in complete silence, avoiding eye contact, and with little bodily movement, simply being the third-party subject of discussion by others. When the conversation between Jim Musgrove and me became animated, she showed such little reaction that the whole scenario had the air of fierce bidding over an inanimate object at an auction.

He prodded the sheets of papers lying on the desk, St. James' Epistle to the Neurologists, Chapter 14. "You can read all about it there."

Of course, I felt sympathy for Mrs. Musgrove and would wish that she did not have any seizures at all. But she had them only once every two months and they were really quite mild, lasting for only one to two minutes with just a little stiffening of the body. She did not have the violent convulsions and falling to the ground that most people associate with epilepsy. The other problem was that she was completely intolerant of all medications that we tried.

"Well, we could increase the dose of her tablets but we tried that before and she became dizzy and dopey. That does not mean that she would get the same side effects now," I said more with optimism than realism "but there is obviously a risk."

"I know, I know," said Mr. Musgrove, shaking his head.

"She is just tolerating her present treatment. We could change to another treatment but we have tried three other medications in the past and all of them made her dopey" I explained.

"I know, I know," said Mr. Musgrove, shaking his head.

"I think I must have a sensitive brain," interjected Mrs. Musgrove in her unique resigned tone, "but I think I am quite a strong person really."

By now, my clinic was running fifteen minutes late. I went over the options again, keeping things as they were and accepting that at least the seizures were relatively mild and infrequent, increasing the dose of her present treatment or changing to another. After a few pauses broken by heavy expiratory gasps, Mr. Musgrove said, "I think we had better stay as we are."

"I think so", said Mrs. Musgrove.

The consultation ended and we decided to review the situation in three months' time. I did not voice the possibility of leaving the appointment open and having her come back only if things changed, on the grounds that the situation had been essentially similar for several years, because I did not have the time.

Outpatient clinics provide a much greater cross-section of illness than hospital admissions because the latter are either emergencies or people who have been selected for further investigation. People also get better, which may be one reason why a proportion of booked patients at every clinic fail to attend, DNAs or "did not attend", as they are known. The DNA rate varies enormously but can be as high as thirty percent. Interestingly, the rate always goes up during the period leading up to Christmas, presumably because the pressure of catering for the in-laws and the building of little Johnny's flat-packed trampoline afford no time to be ill. I once thought that a stress-free, profitable occupation would be to run a private clinic that specialises in DNAs. Appointments could be put at one-minute intervals; a modest charge could be made for each failed attendance; and all the letters to the general practitioner would be the same: "Your patient failed to attend his/her appointment for the clinic today." A nice little earner, really.

At twelve o' clock that day, as I felt like winding down during the last hour before lunch, I had one more new patient to see. I called in Mrs. Dixon, who was a thirty-two-year-old, slim, attractive, well-dressed woman with thick, shiny blonde hair, flowing gently just onto her shoulders. Despite her attractive well-groomed appearance, there was something not quite right about her. She hardly smiled and her face showed little spontaneous movement. She barely altered her position throughout the whole of the consultation.

My initial impression was that she might be depressed, a thought which filled me with some selfish anxiety because I knew that it can be difficult to unravel symptoms due to depression from those due to physical disease. People with depression or other psychological problems do not necessarily just feel bad in their mind but they also develop real physical symptoms that do not have a physical basis.

She told me that she had developed pins and needles in her feet approximately six weeks previously but herself admitted that she thought they might be caused by stress. It didn't take long to find out why. Twelve weeks before, her father had died suddenly. She was emotionally very close to him and took his death very badly such that she had to take sick leave from work. During the two weeks that she was away from work, her manager effected a reorganisation of the department that had been planned for several months and took the opportunity to make her redundant. She believed that the reorganisation was an excuse to dismiss her because they had not got on well together for some time and her sick leave had acted as the final straw for the manager. She was contemplating taking the matter to an industrial tribunal but realised that she would not be paid in the interim, even if her application was successful, and she and her husband would be dependent for the foreseeable future on one instead of two incomes. Six weeks before my consultation, her husband was killed in a car crash.

She had been in very good health before all this. She did not smoke or drink excessively and went running in her local woods at least three times each week. The only problem she had had, and that was not really severe, was that she had blurred vision in one eye for a few weeks about four years previously. She had no other symptoms apart from the pins and needles.

It seemed most likely that her symptoms were stress-induced but I explained that it was necessary to carry out a neurological examination to ensure that there were no signs of physical disease. I went through all the routine tests, including movement of the eyes, visual acuity, strength and coordination and found nothing wrong. However, when it came to testing the reflexes, it was obvious things were not right. Reflexes are enlisted by tapping a muscle tendon gently with a rubber hammer, which results in contraction of the muscle and jerking of the limb, as in the familiar knee jerk. The reflexes in both legs were much brisker than those in the arms. That in itself is not definitely abnormal but two further reflex tests confirmed the problem. I pulled the foot upwards at the ankle using the palm of my hand against her sole. This manoeuvre does not usually produce much in the way of a reaction but, in her case, the foot went into rhythmic up-and-down movements as long as I kept the pressure on her sole, a phenomenon known as clonus. For the second test, I stroked the sole of the foot gently with a key. The reflex reaction is usually for the big toe to move downwards but, in her case, it moved upwards towards the face. Both of these signs indicated definite damage to the nerves that travel down through the spinal cord to the legs and showed that she very probably had something wrong with the spinal cord to cause those reflex changes and also to explain the pins and needles in the feet.

And then something registered in my mind that would have been obvious to someone with more experience. The loss of vision that she had in one eye a few years previously was probably optic neuritis, a warning of a potential future neurological disorder. It was clear that, over a period of twelve weeks, not only had she lost her father, husband and job, but she had also developed multiple sclerosis.

One week later, almost to the day, I received a telephone call as the registrar on call. The general practitioner explained that he had a twenty-three-year-old female patient who had developed numbness in both feet about three days previously. The symptoms had spread up both legs since the onset and now she was incapable of walking. Fresh from my recent learning exercise, I arranged for her to be admitted to the Neurology Ward as an emergency and called my senior house officer, John Barton, to let me know when she arrived.

John finally called me at 11 p.m., fortunately before I had gone to bed. He told me that he had confirmed the history given by the GP and had had a brief look at the patient to find fairly rapidly that she was indeed incapable of walking. I went straight away to the hospital.

On the way to the bedside, John gave me some further details, including that there seemed to be nothing of relevance in the past history and the patient had been in generally good health until this episode. She was a medical student who had just begun her second year of clinical studies.

We carried out a routine detailed neurological examination and found nothing wrong around the head or arms. When we examined the legs, the most obvious finding was that she could only lift the legs about three inches off the bed and said that the muscles were too weak to do anymore. I began to realise that we had not advanced by one jot the GP's diagnosis of subacute weakness of both legs. We tried for something a little more erudite.

Further testing showed that there was no abnormal stiffness in the muscles and the reflexes were normal. In fact, there was nothing abnormal at all to find except the weaknesss and even that was variable. Although she could not lift either leg off the bed, she could push each leg up against my hand with reasonable power. If I lifted the leg in the air and let go, there was a momentary pause before the leg crashed on to the bed, indicating that the muscles had temporarily held the leg satisfactorily high in the air. These were very odd features.

I did not want to make the same mistake that I had done with Mrs. Dixon one week before but I had to see what this lady was capable of doing with support. With John's help, I got her on to her feet. As we held her by the arms, one of us on each side, her legs crumpled beneath her. With encouragement, however, the leg muscles started to contract and she adopted a bouncing manoeuvre like a puppet on a string. Twenty minutes later, we had her walking down the ward.

We did further tests over the next few days but found no evidence of neurological disease. A psychiatrist established that she was under considerable stress in her medical studies because she could not avoid believing that she was going to contract every new condition that she saw. She had physical symptoms resulting from purely psychological causes.

I have found it easier to identify with the characters who verge upon hysteria, who were frightened of life, who were desperate to reach out to another person. But these seemingly fragile people are the strong people really. Tennessee Williams

Pain is real when you get other people to believe in it. If no one believes in it but you, your pain is madness or hysteria. Naomi Wolf

Jackie had stayed in Oxford during the eighteen months that I was away. By now, she was a staff nurse on the Coronary Care Unit, a job that mostly involved sitting staring at a monitor that displayed the pulse, blood pressure and electrical activity of the heart, or lack thereof, depending upon the current health of the patient. There were usually four of these young women huddled around the screen at any one time, all wearing the dark brown uniform of the staff nurse grade and refusing to smile. It was hard not to draw analogies with bees round a honey pot. Coronary Care Unit nurses have a fearsome reputation because their skills in drawing back patients from the jaws of death when the heartbeat develops a potentially fatal abnormality of rhythm fit them with a life-or-death persona, coupled with an air of intolerance. Newly qualified house officers are the favourite prey of these raptors. Many is the young doctor called to the Coronary Care Unit to deal with an abnormality of heart rhythm in one of the patients to be thrown an ECG strip by four austere ladies in brown with the direction to tell them the nature of the abnormality and what is going to be done about it. The welfare of the patient ultimately requires them to ease the poor medic's state of agitated burbling by providing the answer.

I was seldom called to the Coronary Care Unit in those days because it did not have much to do with neurology so I cannot say whether Jackie behaved in that way or not but somehow I cannot see it. At the very least, I expect she would be the one who first put the houseman out of his misery.

I don't know what she had done or who she had been with while I was away because, even though we had spoken on the telephone fairly regularly, she had never volunteered any information and I did not want to ask. We had coffee together from time to time and met over lunch in the hospital cafeteria, usually more by accident than design. Fate had not thrown us constantly together in the way that it had eighteen months earlier. We were emotionally close but increasingly obviously had different lives - "like a brother and sister" may be a cliche but nonetheless true.

One day she told me that she had decided to leave Oxford to join the Army as a nurse. When we went out for lunch to say goodbye, I asked her if she thought we should have got married.

"No," she said simply.

"Why not?" I asked.

"I just don't think we should."

"Wouldn't you have enjoyed it?" I asked naively.

"Probably very much but I still don't think we should."

As promised, she wrote to me a few weeks later but I did not reply. There was no deliberate reason not to do so but something stopped me, possibly the fact that she told me that she was surrounded by lots of gorgeous men. There were no more letters and I have not seen or heard of her since.

I think of her often and hope whoever she's met will be fully aware of how precious she is.   Bob Dylan "Ballad in Plain D"

Patients come in all shapes and sizes, literally and metaphorically. Not surprising, perhaps, because, on the whole, they represent a cross-section of society. It is amazing how difficult it is to get people to change their physical and mental habits, even if it is to their advantage.

Obese people tend to present to clinics dealing with heart disease, high blood pressure and diabetes. Appeals to lose weight for their own sake are met with a variety of responses:

"I've always been big. My mother and sisters are big."

"I tried and I can't."

"Well, I know somebody half my weight and they still got diabetes."

"I just like my food."

Some doctors go to extreme lengths to get their patients to lose weight. I knew one consultant who told his overweight patients "There were no fat people in the Belsen concentration camp." Maybe he got away with it because he was Jewish.   But I have some sympathy with the patients' responses. It is not the responsibility of the doctor to dictate how someone should live but they do need to point out the risks of the particular lifestyle. I had a patient who had been sent from another consultant for a second opinion on the reason that he had developed double vision. None of the tests had provided the answer but routine blood tests had shown abnormal liver tests, almost certainly because the gentleman's main recreational pursuit was alcohol ingestion. I happened to mention the test results, as previous consultants had done, and he admitted that he drank to excess but chose to do so because he enjoyed it. The abnormal liver function tests were not going to put him off.

He added, "You doctors are an interesting lot. I come to see you about a problem with my eyes and get the response 'I've no idea what's wrong with your eyes but I recognise a dodgy liver when I seen one.'" So maybe the spherical suet pudding who likes their food should be allowed to continue liking their food, food and yet more food, provided they understand the risks attached.

By the way, the claim that it is impossible to lose weight might just be correct. I had always thought that a person could not possibly be so large without eating constantly throughout the day unless there was something physically wrong with their metabolism. I have seen a lot of very large people walking into the local swimming pool but have never seen any of them carrying burgers or sandwiches at the time. I doubt that it is original, but I had a thought that the problem might be due to a virus. Low and behold, in 2007, Professor Richard Atkinson, building on work by Dr.

Nihi Dhurandhar in 1992, found evidence to support infection by the virus Ad36 as a cause of obesity.

But it is the different personalities of people that make medicine at once fascinating and frustrating.

It has often been said that the most important part of medical assessment is the taking of the history, that is the patient's account of the nature of the symptoms and how they unravel over time. It may be that this notion has been particularly nurtured by doctors who cannot be bothered to examine patients but there is little doubt that there is some truth in it. It is important not to ask leading questions because some people will agree with everything suggested by the doctor because of awe, anxiety, desire to help or simply not listening. Unfortunately, this reluctance to pin down the patient verbally can lead to major difficulties in obtaining necessary information. A fly on the wall helpfully recorded this conversation for me:

> "When did the headaches first start?"
>
> "About the time of my sister's wedding."
>
> "When was your sister's wedding?"
>
> "Just before the headaches started."
>
> "How long ago was that?"
>
> "Oh, I don't know really."
>
> "Well, was it months or years?"
>
> "Not years, oh no!"
>
> "Was it less than a month?"

"Oh no, it was longer than that!"

"So it was several months ago?"

"If you say so, I suppose it must have been."

"I know it is difficult to describe headaches but what sort of pain is it? What do you feel in your head?"

"Terrible."

"Yes, but is it a throbbing, tightness, stabbing or what?"

"Yes."

"Which?"

"It's just awful. I've got it now."

"Did anything unusual happen at the wedding?"

"She had four pageboys, which I thought was a bit unusual."

"No, I mean anything that you think might have caused the headache."

"I don't see her much now because they went to live in Australia."

Chloe Critchley posed a different problem for the history taker. It was not so much that she failed to answer the questions in whatever format they were posed but her answers were so mundane as to have virtually no meaning.

"How are you today?"

"Can't complain."

"How have you been since your last appointment?"

"Well, a bit up and down I suppose."

"Overall, have you been better or worse?"

"You win some, you lose some."

"Are you still getting migraines?"

"Well, what goes around comes around, after all."

"Are they getting you down?"

"Worse things have happened at sea."

"How often are you getting them now?"

"Once, twice, three times a month who knows, even I don't know everything!"

"How much are they affecting your life? How much time are you having to take off work?"

"I like work it fascinates me. I can sit and look at it for hours. I think that is a famous quote" she said laughing. "I do what I can."

"Are you happy with your present treatment? Would you like to try something else?"

"Better the devil you know ..."

And so it went on.

I ended up calling her Cliché Critchley although not to her face, of course. There is a condition caused by a problem with part of the brain at the front that leads people to make repeated silly jokes, often out of context. I wondered whether I had found something similar in Cliché Critchley and wondered whether I should persuade her to have a brain scan. But, I pondered, how was I going to explain to her the reason for this? After all, she didn't have a definite problem and I had no desire to give the neo-fascist impression that I thought that she was so mad that she ought to undergo investigation. I decided it was just her personality and left it at that.

Most people of course, answer questions well and to the best of their memory. Indeed, the taking of the history should not really be a grilling of the patient by the doctor but more a conversation in which the patient is allowed to give an account of their symptoms freely with prompts where necessary by the doctor. Some people are remarkably clear. Occasionally, the answers can be so precise as to stretch the credibility that a person can have a memory that good. Jack Taverner was one such person. He had developed tingling in the hands and feet with some loss of dexterity.

"When did the trouble start?"

"May 17, 1978."

"That's very precise. Did something special happen that day?"

"No, I just remember it."

"What happened then?"

"I got tingling in the fingers of the left hand except the ring finger and in the right hand except the middle finger."

"And when did you start having difficulty in using your hands?"

"Eight weeks and four days later."

"Have you dropped things from your hands?"

"Yes, five times."

"When was the last time?"

"February 6, 1979."

I wondered whether he was making it up but I had no way of knowing. Some years later, I came across a similar pattern of behaviour whilst doing some research on memory. The test involved giving the subject a cue word such as "apple" and asking them to recount a memory from their own life, however trivial, connected with that word. Again, I observed the same pattern of extremely precise answers from one subject to the extent that it was virtually beyond one's imagination how the memory could be so good. Unlike Mr. Taverner, however, on this occasion I had the opportunity to ask the same questions the following day as part of the test procedure. He gave exactly the same answers. Thus, either the answers were true or he had remembered on the second day the answers that he had given on the first day. The latter seemed very unlikely because he was not warned that he would be asked the questions the following day and again his memory would have to be remarkable to remember such detail.

I concluded that he and Mr. Taverner had an extremely precise memory for detail. The difference between the two patients was that the man on whom I was carrying out the memory research had had a brain injury. It was fascinating to think that somehow damage to a particular part of the brain had improved rather than compromised particular aspects of memory. I was reminded of the person with high-functioning autism who can learn large quantities of unconnected information, such as a telephone directory, a feat that is beyond the capability of most ordinary people. Once again, I wondered whether I should have carried out a brain scan on Mr. Taverner.

But what physician has not had patients who don't make any sense at all? To tell the truth, they're our stock-in-trade. We talk and write about the ones we can make sense of.
Walker Percy

Chapter 6: Inspection

Pluck the ripe and ready and leave the rest to the whims of the tree.

I was in the third year of my registrar job and looking forward to a post of senior registrar. Appointment to the position of senior registrar provided entry to a completely different ball game from the earlier junior posts. The pyramidal structure of appointment, whereby there were more applicants than posts available, largely ceased at senior registrar level. At that point, one could be reasonably assured of a consultant post although, precisely when and where, remained totally uncertain. In neurology, the almost universal location of the departments in major cities provided some comfort because most offered a reasonable standard of living. For other specialities, however, such as general medicine or general surgery, the senior registrar may well gain a post as consultant but it could be in Lower-Bogden-by-The-Sewer, a domicile which might not have been the major aspiration of a surgeon-in-development. There was also a worry that a minority of senior registrars ended up as permanent lackeys to their consultants. Remember Donald, who was the senior registrar to Mr. Potts when I was a student, and portrayed a persona of one permanently suppressed into a life of subservient flagellation. I do not know if he ever got a job as a consultant. If not, he probably ended up as a butler or manservant in some equivalent of an early twentieth-century grand house whose main qualification that set him apart from others on appointment was his ability to operate on the rest of the domestic staff.

I applied for two jobs without success, one at Guy's Hospital and one at Bart's Hospital, both in London, and both very prestigious teaching hospitals. It was obvious which of the candidates for those jobs would ultimately get the job, such was the power of the pre-interview bush telegraph in those days. The expected victor at the Guy's interview was indeed appointed despite his habit prior to the interview of vociferously voicing his opinions on the qualities, or lack thereof, of the consultants for whom he would ultimately work if appointed.

So much seemed to have been decided in advance of the interview that one wondered, with some justification, whether the interview was of any deciding value at all. I was reminded of my time as a house officer in Bath, when a senior house officer there applied for a job at a famous teaching hospital in London to find himself amongst five other selected candidates, all of whom, unlike him, had qualified from the hospital. He realised that he was the cannon fodder, the token candidate, from a district general hospital, who stood practically no chance of gaining the appointment. At the end of the interview formalities, he was invited to ask if there was anything about the job that was not clear to him. He asked, "Is this job recognised for higher professional training?", a question which must have been superfluous for an organisation with such recognition. The interviewers bumbled, almost certainly because such a challenge to their authority had never been placed. "Er, er, I think it must be," replied the chairman of the interviewing panel. "Well, yes, I am certain," he continued and, turning to his fellow interviewers for support, terminated the discussion and the immediate future prospects of my friend with the putdown, "I suggest you check with Personnel, if and when you are appointed." Needless to say, he wasn't.

It was Thursday, 4 March 1980, the day of the senior registrar interviews at Oxford. Nicholas Martin, the previous incumbent, had just been appointed to a consultant post in Reading, forty miles from Oxford, with two sessions (half days) in Oxford. There was an increasing tendency to move a consultant's main base away from the teaching centre to one of the district hospitals in the region, ostensibly to make life easier for patients who previously may have had to travel up to sixty miles to see a consultant. Another reason, I have no doubt, is that the expansion in the consultant base that was taking place around that time could never be accommodated in the main regional centre because there simply wasn't enough space. Established consultants were not all that willing to share offices or beds (for the patients, that is). For many new appointees, the development was a treat because they didn't have to negotiate with difficult neurological colleagues except for two half days per week; they were essentially their own boss in the district general hospital and they could live in the country, which, for Nick at least, was a delight. Nick's sessions in Oxford were also largely academic so he could spend the time sitting in on grand rounds and lectures in lofty silence, interrupted only by the occasional comment, uttered with the indifference of someone who doesn't really need to be there at all.

Nick kept goats, chickens and horses. He once responded to the then popular habit of consultants of describing a clinical situation as "as clear as a barn door" or "barn door obvious" by pointing out that many of them would probably not recognise a barn door if they saw one.

I waited patiently outside the interview room for my turn to be interrogated. No doubt my feelings were similar in many ways to those of anyone waiting for the chance to get a job that is at once important and desirable. But there always seemed to me something a bit special about medical interviews.

Rightly or wrongly, it was difficult to escape the conclusion that the assessment would consider attributes that were not necessarily so much concerned with being a good neurologist as with being a good consultant colleague - and that is not the same thing. Anyway, for whatever reason, on that day I had a lot of sympathy with the inmates of Death Row, knowing not if, but when, my run of medical good fortune would finally end.

I was reminded of my undergraduate interview at Oxford fourteen years earlier because I was confronted by a semicircle of consultants and asked to sit in a chair roughly at the point of the centre of the circle. When I later became a consultant, and carried out interviews, I developed a retrospective sympathy for my interviewers because I realised that, beyond the obvious, it is difficult to think of something to ask. Often one of the previous questioners unwittingly steals the choice question that you have kept patiently ready to pose when your turn came.

I should have guessed as much then when one of them asked me what single measure I would take as Chief Medical Officer to improve the health of the nation. Instead of feeling irritated that he seemed not to know that this was an interview for senior registrar and not the most senior medical adviser to the government, I should have realised that his planned question "Why do you want this job?" had been asked five minutes earlier.

All went well, having given good ripostes to the early challenges, until approximately half way through the interview when I suddenly felt a real physical draining of energy, spreading down from my head to my feet. All I wanted to do was to go to sleep but I thought that a little unwise. I held on but have no idea what I said and probably was equally unclear even at the time. The last two consultants came to my rescue: "No questions." I expect they were totally bored or as tired as I was but perhaps also a little brave because they both received brief disapproving sideways glances from their colleagues.

No matter: the smiles on all their faces when I was called back in were a transformation. I had successfully completed the Trial by Psychological Destruction to become Senior Registrar.

Two days later, I was back in clinic. But – not as Registrar, but as Senior Registrar Elect! Not that it made a blind bit of difference. The nurses, reception staff, physiotherapists and most certainly the patients were unlikely to change their attitude just because some poxy doctor had made a good career move, even if they knew about it (which they didn't). Never mind; I felt better and a little sorry for all these people who failed to appreciate how, by just one interview, my skills as a doctor had taken A Great Leap Forward.

Chapter 7: Foreign varieties

If the grass seems greener on the other side of the hill, it is probably a different species.

Some qualifications are essential to becoming a consultant physician. For a start, it helps a lot to have a medical degree but, on top of that, Membership of the Royal College of Physicians is a sine qua non. Then, there are the qualifications that are *desirable* but not *essential*, such as a past job in research, properties that provide distinction from competitors with equivalent basic skills. In principle, anything that allows your CV to stand out from the rest will do, provided it is reasonably moral.

Unfortunately, the more people collect these distinguishing badges, the less they distinguish. When every applicant has a previous research job listed on their CV, something else has to be found to provide that "little extra". Life events of increasingly dubious relevance become incorporated into assessment criteria. An Oxbridge blue in rowing may not be an obvious asset for a senior doctor but it will, if you choose so to argue, help produce a more fulfilled personality and hence a better doctor. Hmmmm. It probably also helps if you intend to specialise in the management of rowing injuries.

One popular desirable but not essential qualification in the early 1980s was the BTA (Been To America). I cannot recall now the post hoc rationalisation that led to the inclusion of this particular experience in the list of desirable attributes, probably because the logic of it was largely irrelevant: the important point was that, at some point, it had proven useful as an arbitrary indicator to distinguish candidates and therefore later became a desirable property for a candidate in the gaining of points against one's competitors. As long as the badge was still deemed desirable, it continued to distinguish. Only when the majority of applicants had collected this particular badge was it necessary to find some other and then, of course, the BTA, like all others, could be removed from the desirable list, only to return when nobody bothered doing it anymore because it provided no tangible career benefit. Such considerations were even more important if there was the intention of working in a particular city, as opposed to any that proved sufficiently magnanimous to offer employment.

On Friday, 14 January 1983, my wife and two-year-old daughter waited in a queue at Heathrow Airport, ready to entrust our six suitcases, representing a mobile embodiment of our current life, to the check-in clerk. Actually, to be strictly accurate, my wife and I waited and my daughter waited intermittently. Soon we would be following in the footsteps of the Pilgrim Fathers to the Land of the Free to settle like them on the eastern seaboard at a place now called Boston. The trip was no doubt essentially similar to theirs except in minor detail, such as a jet airliner, hotel on arrival and alcoholic drinks en route. (Dear Reader, I have not troubled you with the details of the courtship and marriage of my lovely wife and the arrival of my beautiful daughter. Suffice it to say for the purposes of this account that both were acquired by fairly traditional means.)

William Jackson, my American mentor-to-be, was to meet us at the airport and take us to the Holiday Inn in Somerville, which we had booked before departure. When we spoke on the telephone before departure, he told me he had never heard such a classic English accent. I wondered whether to reciprocate by praising his American accent but felt uncomfortable with the notion that this was a compliment. I am glad I didn't because I was reliably informed some months later (by an American) that Americans don't have an accent; but the English do. Strange, isn't it, how normality becomes defined from one's own perspective? Incidentally, North America is probably the only English-speaking region whose inhabitants make no distinction in the pronunciation of Mary, merry and marry (although this does not apply to Boston).

I would recognise Will, he told me, because he had no facial hair and would be wearing blue jeans. As these features were presumably identified in order to distinguish him from the crowd, I pondered on the appearance of all the other Bostonians: besuited and bearded?

I did not know then that "blue jeans" are to the US what "jeans" are to the UK so I told him that I too lacked facial hair and would probably be wearing green jeans. I expect he thought I was taking the piss. Perhaps, however, he knew more English than I did American because, on arrival at the airport, he strode forward, wearing blue jeans and lacking facial hair, to greet us with an air of recognition similar to that bestowed when meeting a long-lost friend.

His face fell only twice. Once was at the realisation that his station wagon was to accommodate two adults, a child and six suitcases as well as himself. (I thought of offering to leave the child behind but felt this might label me as a negligent parent.) The second was when he learnt that our hotel was in Somerville. I still don't know whether it was the distance from the airport that bothered him or the low tone of the neighbourhood. I discovered later that Bostonians pride themselves on being of original American stock (apart from the native Americans, that is) and convey an impression, deliberate or otherwise, of class-consciousness. Maybe Somerville was a place that the Jacksons simply do not visit - *because that's how it is*. But the Bostonians are also friendly. And they have a remarkable capacity to dissociate the personal from the professional. More than once have I heard an employee being dismissed, only to be invited by the same person to a party a few minutes later. Will was very much like that. He drove us to Somerville without complaint.

I suspected that any apartment that we could afford in downtown Boston would be a cockroach nest so we chose to rent in a small town called Acton, twenty miles out. Acton was mostly one street, lined by single-storey shops, but it had everything required, including an Italian restaurant, liquor store and guitar school. The apartment building grounds also included a swimming pool, supervised by an attractive young female lifeguard, who befriended my daughter (but not me). We rented furniture, raided the local store for crockery and cutlery, used sheets as curtains and were thereby mostly set up.

Except for transport. Maintenance work was underway on the railway line to North Station, causing disruption to a direct journey from home to Boston, where I would work each day. There seemed little choice but to buy a car.

The man in the used-car lot was short but his hair was long and he sported a moustache that seemed too big for him in general and his face in particular. The effect was exemplified by his lack of facial movement, his lips being held clamped together in the guise of someone holding total contempt for everything and everyone around him.

There seemed no question of considering any car that he had not personally selected for us. His descriptions were all brief and largely paraphrases of each other.

"Chevrolet. Three litre. 1973. Fifteen hundred bucks. A beauty," or something very similar.

I was tempted by a geriatric Lincoln Continental 7.5 litre that looked as if it accommodated about eighteen people, all supine, had a suspension similar to a waterbed and did about two and a half miles to the gallon. These cars were icons of past times but rejected by many people on average salaries because of lack of affordability. And that's why I opted for the 1200 c.c. Renault 5. Mr. Disenchanted reacted as if I had ignored his tip of the sure-win rank outsider at the Grand National. However, he agreed to sell the Renault, probably because we were mad English and at least he was making some money.

"Anything else I need?" I asked as the deal was done, my licence was checked and insurance organised, all on the spot.

"Like what?" he growled.

"Road tax."

"Road tax??!!" he blurted, eyes on fire.

"Yes, in the UK, we have to pay road tax."

"Well, don't mention it here or someone'll sure think about it." That was the longest sentence he produced over the course of one and a half hours.

I drove away, pleased at having legally avoided road tax and a little proud at having chosen a European car, even though it had about a quarter of the seating, power and comfort of the Lincoln and none of the panache. At least, I wouldn't have to fill up with fuel every twenty miles.

An American is a man with two arms and four wheels.
A Chinese child

Three days later was to be my first full day in Boston. With a clinical and research fellowship, I was to divide my time between seeing patients at the Massachusetts General Hospital and doing research at Massachusetts Institute of Technology. Will's specialities within neurology were memory and movement disorders, mostly Alzheimer's disease and Parkinson's disease so, perhaps not surprisingly, these were the patients I saw. Just a few months earlier, I had had to take and pass the Visa Qualifying Examination (VQE), which tested my knowledge in all the basic subjects of the medical course, including specialities such as gynaecology that I had not visited, at least in a professional capacity, since my student days. Fresh from the mind-broadening experience of yet another exam, I felt a little disappointed at having now to restrict my intellectual energy to subspecialities of neurology. I could easily have thrown in a few vaginal examinations along the way.

Apart from having to satisfy the American authorities that I was proficient in medical areas with which I was never to have any dealings, I was also required to demonstrate my linguistic skills by taking an English test as part of the VQE. It seemed a very odd requirement until a large American psychiatrist explained to me later that it was really a test in American. I still felt sure that American was an easier language to learn for an English speaker than French, in which I had had no testing when I worked in a Parisian hospital for a few months, four years earlier. By the way, the VQE application form required identification of nationality at three different times of life: birth, on entering medical school and on leaving medical school. I am still not sure whom that was supposed to catch.

Health care in the United States is mostly operated by the private sector and funded by insurance companies but many people are uninsured and the problem is getting worse. A US Census Bureau report indicates that about thirty million people or roughly thirteen percent of the population had no health insurance in 1987, three years after I was there, and the first year that data were collected. Interestingly, by 2009, the figure had increased to 50.7 million or 16.7 percent of the population. Hinnelstein and colleagues, reporting in the American Journal of Medicine, showed that 62.1 percent of all bankruptcies in 2007 were medically related, either because of loss of income due to illness or having to pay medical bills. In 1981 the figure was eight percent. The share of bankruptcies related to medical problems had increased by 49.6 percent from 2001. Ninety-two percent of medical debtors had medical debts over five thousand dollars or ten percent of pretax family income. The average medical debt for uninsured people in 2007 was nearly twenty-seven thousand dollars.

Financial ruin from medical bills is almost exclusively an American disease. Roul Turley

Ellie May lived in a rented apartment of our building with her husband and daughter, Lori. Mom and Dad were in their early twenties; Lori was aged four. Ellie May did not have a job; the current Dad gained just enough income from labouring jobs to pay the rent, feed the family and cover other household costs. But it would all have been a lot easier if they were not saddled with a debt for fifteen thousand dollars for medical costs related to an accident he had at work two years earlier. The nature of his work did not provide for any employment-related insurance and they could not afford to pay premiums themselves. All they could now manage was to pay the interest on the loan; there was not the remotest chance of their ever paying off the capital sum. Quite what they would do if they were to become ill in the future is, as they say, not at all clear. Some respite existed in the form of Medicare, a Government programme, if they were lucky enough to reach the age of sixty-five, and by Medicaid if they could engineer their poverty to combine with one of the other criteria of the programme, such as disability. So, hey, all was not lost.

I recently became a Christian Scientist. It was the only health plan I could afford. Betsy Salkind

The Mass General, where I was to work, was founded in 1811 and is the third oldest general hospital in the United States (the other two are probably the Bellevue Hospital and the Presbyterian Hospital, both in New York). It is considered to be one of the top three hospitals in the US. Its number one ranking in psychiatry and location in Fruit Street are probably coincidences. It has more than two hundred thousand employees and public parking rates currently around forty dollars per day. So it is successful in many ways.

There was a rule, I assume unwritten, concerning dress code at the Mass General. Round about the time that man was coming down from the trees and starting to make tools that would at first be used for skinning antelopes but later for opening each other's skulls, someone thought it would be cute if all consultants dressed in blue and white striped suits. It must have made a lovely sight, worthy of any male catwalk, to see five or six consultants, all identically dressed in blue and white stripes, walking towards you in conversation down the hallowed corridors of one of the most famous hospitals in America. I never did learn whether this habit was common to all specialities or peculiar to neurology but I imagine it depended on the intensity of self-delusion in sartorial elegance of the speciality concerned.

Except for one or two die-hards, the staff had sadly largely abandoned the dress by the time I arrived in Boston, possibly because it had a passing resemblance to a prisoner-of-war uniform. But I am pleased that the Hospital still has an interest in fashion. The following is the current dress code, and associated economic policy, for volunteers:

"Volunteers who are in hospital assignments are required to wear a volunteer jacket or polo shirt. The jacket is secured with a refundable $15 deposit. The polo shirt is purchased for $15. Each volunteer is responsible for keeping his or her own jacket or shirt clean and bringing it to volunteer each week."

"Once you have left your position as a volunteer, you have 90 days to return your jacket and receive your original $15 deposit. If the jacket is clean, you will receive a full refund of $15. If the jacket is soiled, the deposit will be reduced to $10 to cover the cost of cleaning the jacket. If you return the jacket beyond 90 days, we will be unable to refund the deposit but are happy to accept the jacket back for use in the program. We are unable to refund any money for the polo shirts."

"Dress code prohibits the wearing of blue jeans, sweatpants, exercise pants, shorts, hats, sunglasses, T-shirts and open-toed shoes."

One wonders at the financial implications of returning a soiled jacket after ninety days. Would you be charged five dollars simply to deposit the jacket at the Hospital? The Charles River would be cheaper.

On the day of my first drive into Boston, it started to snow. My impression of the USA is that it has more of everything: more land, more mountains, more corn, more coke, more riches, more poverty. And more weather. The sun doesn't just shine; it blazes. The wind doesn't just blow; it makes tornados. And the snow makes British snow scenes look like one of those glass bowls filled with water and containing an endearing scene in plastic that becomes coated in the gentlest of snow showers when the bowl is inverted.

The snow came down in flakes the size of plates, all perfectly vertically, and gathered on the road within minutes. Sensing something bigger than I might have been able to handle, I called in at the filling station on the edge of Acton.

"Do you think I will make it into Boston this morning," I asked.

"Mebbee," replied the attendant.

"Do you think I will make it back this evening?"

"Mebbee not."

I went home and tried again when the snow had cleared about four months later. Well, I exaggerate, but there was a four months' stay of the snow, not necessarily still falling from the skies but gradually compacting by the roadside and changing by degrees from a virginal white to a dirty grey.

On Monday mornings, I attended the Memory Disorders Clinic where I would see a selection of new patients, assuming they remembered to attend. The clinic had dual roles: one clinical, to diagnose, treat and otherwise manage the patient; the other research, to spot cases that may be suitable for drug trials. The commonest cause of serious memory loss is Alzheimer's disease for which there were, and still are, few useful treatments. Discovery of a drug that was effective in reversing memory loss or preventing further deterioration would be like gold dust, metaphorically and, for the pharmaceutical company at least, literally.

Will was involved in research on two drugs at the time. The criteria for entry into the two trials were slightly different, so patients had to be mentally classified on assessment not only into trial or no trial but also trial one or trial two. Combining these thoughts simultaneously with ones devoted towards care of the patient could produce conflicts of interest. But since there was no useful drug available, entry into a drug trial was probably the patient's best option.

I called my first patient, Vernon Gruber, a white male aged seventy-three who attended with his wife. After the usual introductions, I started on the history.

"What is it that has brought you to see me?" Fortunately, he didn't say "an ambulance" as one patient did a few months later.

"It's his memory," said Mrs. Gruber. "It's awful."

"Do you agree, Mr. Gruber?"

"Suppose so. I can't remember."

"How long has it been a problem?"

"I forget right now," he said. But Mrs. Gruber was keen to enlighten me.

"Months. He just doesn't try. The son-of a-bitch does it on purpose."

"How do you know?"

"I haven't lived with him for thirty-five years without knowing something about him."

I pondered quite why she had stuck out the thirty-five years when she seemed to dislike him so much but I knew he had changed and her anger reflected her anxiety.

"He's not the same guy, not at all", she said more quietly and that summed up her problem.

And then she started to cry. There is a sweet side to the dragon, I thought. It's heartbreaking to see a slow relentless decay of memory in a loved one. But she soon clarified:

"I am having to do everything now – all the chores, going to the store, cleaning the yard. And I am not well myself."

"Who did it all before?"

"Well, he did!" she exclaimed, as if I had asked a silly question (and, given what I knew of this couple so far, probably had).

"You've got to do something, doc. I am going to end up really ill, if it carries on like this."

I went through the rest of the history, did a physical examination and a brief memory test, identified him as a trial two candidate and turned my attention back to her. Out of normal courtesy, I spoke directly to him but knew he was not taking it in and so framed my discussion for her ears.

The most likely diagnosis was Alzheimer's disease I explained but usually the memory loss occurs much more slowly.

"Well, he has been like it for years," she said.

"I thought you said months."

"Well, he has been like this for months but he has not been right for years."

"In what way?"

"Bad memory."

There are times in medicine when you realise that some behaviours defy a rationale explanation and this was one of them. I gave up aiming for historical precision because I felt that I too would end up really ill if it carries on like this.

He agreed to undergo further tests and so did she – on him, that is. In truth, he wasn't really fit to give informed consent and we needed her on board if we were going to do anything to even try and help – which probably meant trial two.

The routine was to meet next to Will's office after each clinic to discuss the cases. The venue was a seminar room but it looked more like a boardroom and, on the face of it, had precious little to do with medicine. In attendance were John, a psychiatrist, the psychology research team from MIT, two research fellows including me, a statistician and a research secretary. It's serious stuff dealing with these dementia cases, let me tell you! Most of the people present said nothing. Will would ask one of the research fellows to give details of the next case which would prompt what might loosely be called "discussion", usually consisting of a single statement from Will, "So a trial one player then?" (To be strictly accurate, there were two variants of this question because it could concern trial two instead.) The statistician in particular never, to my knowledge, said anything at all but spent the whole time looking depressed, maybe with good reason because it is very difficult to do meaningful statistics on cases presented one at a time.

"So will you speak to Mrs. Gruber?"

(Not if I can get away with it.) "Yes, of course" I replied.

After the clinic, we returned to MIT. The journey to and fro was usually carried out on foot over the Longfellow Bridge across the Charles River unless, that is, the city's air pollution reached a level that risked wiping out half of the population. Only once in eighteen months was there an official declaration that the city was effectively uninhabitable outside of a hermetically sealed car or a coffin but, on a number of other summer days, I wished I had been wearing goggles to at least limit the corneal erosions invoked by the airborne acids.

At MIT, I shared an office with two postdoctoral fellows (or postdocs as they are known in the trade). Actually the occupancy was a bit variable. The three of us were fixed tenants but most of the Psychology Department passed through the office at regular intervals, sometimes staying briefly to chat and at other times taking a seat at one of the desks, without invitation, to edit some research paper they were carrying. I suspect every other office in the building was used in the same way. I rationalised that a virtuoso researcher cannot afford the delay between the realisation of some universal truth and arrival back at one's own office for fear that the intellectual gem will be lost. So the only answer is to take temporary root at the point of spiritual dawning in order to record the discovery there and then for the benefit of future humankind. Either that or they were slightly mad – or both.

The principle of the neuropsychology research carried out at MIT was to work out precisely what was wrong with the memory and intellect of someone with damage to a known, specific part of the brain. By implication, the same part of the brain controlled those functions in people without brain damage. The non-damaged group are usually called "normal" but anyone who has looked even slightly closely at most "normal" people will realise that the group probably doesn't exist at all – the whole human race is, to a greater or lesser extent, barmy. But we were dealing with functions, such as memory, that are not usually considered to be major determinants of barminess so members of the "normal" group are more similar in that respect than you might expect.

Damage to specific parts of the brain produces the most extraordinary effects as now any one of thousands of researchers, books and articles around the world will tell you. If it didn't exist, I don't think you could make it up or, if you did, no one would believe you. The amnesic can do everything but remember – an ace at the Daily Telegraph crossword but unable to remember anything about it – or even having done it at all - forty-five seconds after he has put it down. On the whole disabling, but quite handy if you have to spend time with disagreeable relatives; at least you feel good very soon after they have gone away. One amnesic also pointed out to me that you can have great fun going on holiday repeatedly to the same place because each visit seems like a completely novel adventure.

Mrs. Kennedy had visual agnosia. She could see perfectly well but she had selective inability to recognise objects. Ann held up an orange.

"What is that?" she said.

"I don't know," replied Mrs. Kennedy.

"Can you describe it for me?"

"Yes, it is fairly small, round, a bit knobbly over the surface."

"Why don't you hold it?" asked Ann. "Can you tell me anything else?"

"Well, it is fairly soft, you can squeeze it between your fingers."

"What colour is it?"

"Orange."

"Do you know what it is?"

"No."

The aphasic is kind of the opposite. He or she knows what the object is but cannot find the word for it. You can meet aphasics who have difficulty with only one category of object, such as living but not nonliving things. Who knows what may turn up next? Inability to name frozen but not non-frozen food? Green but not red vegetables? Spouse but not mistress? I wouldn't be surprised.

But the best for entertainment value are those with frontal-lobe damage. The frontal lobes of the brain deal with more complex functions, such as planning, judgement, self-control, and, broadly, personality, which are lost or altered by damage to the area.

Mrs. Diamond, for example, had developed frontal-lobe damage when a pickaxe fell from a shelf and penetrated her skull (sorry if you are squeamish). She had agreed to come to a case conference attended by most of the hospital consultants in order to discuss her case and thereby fulfil the worthwhile dual aims of education and acquisition of the necessary number of hours of continuing professional development required to remain in medical practice.

Seated on the front row was Matt Digby, a serious radiologist with glossy grey hair, chubby cheeks and no smile. As Mrs. Diamond entered the room, she glanced briefly at Matt before throwing herself onto his lap, "Aren't you gorgeous?" being the spontaneous explanation of her behaviour. If Matt had been capable of looking even less amused than usual, he would have.

It is no surprise that such people (patients not radiologists) used to be locked away in madhouses but even then doctors were smart enough to know that producing a different form of frontal lobe damage would have the opposite effect, production of a compliant, apathetic individual. Hence was the fashion for frontal lobotomy, which, if pressed for time, could be carried out at the bedside. Insertion of a metal rod up the nose, through the thin bone at the top that separates the nostril from the brain, penetration of the frontal lobe and a few deft spiralling motions of the rod would soon produce the desired effect. And very few complaints afterwards.

After about three months, we had made a few interesting observations that we thought worthy of presentation at a research conference, where scientists from around the world come to disagree with the findings of everyone except their friends. We had been lucky enough to be given a platform presentation, which meant that I, as lead worker on the research, was granted the dubious privilege of standing on a stage giving a slide show to perhaps five hundred cynics in the audience. The time allotted was fifteen minutes. As we worked on the slides and talk, Samuel Bywaters' words repeated themselves in my mind at regular intervals: "To talk for thirty minutes would be easy, but I want you to talk for ten minutes." What do you put in and what do you leave out? I thought of omitting all the results of our experiments and getting the audience to predict the outcome from the background to the research and the methods we used. That would fill fifteen minutes or so but I feared that the voters would fall into only three categories: those who did research that essentially agreed with ours, those who didn't and those who didn't care or were asleep (the latter group was not uncommon at such meetings). People, you see, mostly vote for themselves.

Eventually we had fine-tuned the presentation to fourteen minutes, fifty seconds with fifteen slides and were ready to go.

My first ever research presentation was to be at the annual meeting of the Association of British Neurologists held, on this occasion, in St. John's, Newfoundland, jointly with the Newfoundland Neurological Society. The UK with a population of sixty million had only about two hundred consultant neurologists at that time. Newfoundland, with a population of about half a million, had a lot fewer. I can't remember exactly how many but equally do not remember seeing any of them at the meeting.

My turn was at 10:00 a.m. on the Friday, the third day of the three-day conference. Not a bad time because people tend to be still interested but, with leaving for home easily in their sights, not too aggressive. At 9.00 am that day, I was to be seen, in mounting anxiety, pacing up and down the coastline in my best and only suit explaining the finer points of selective memory loss to a rather kindly looking iceberg in the harbour.

Motives for attending international conferences can be quite varied but you have to be serious about something to travel three thousand miles to attend a meeting populated by people most of whom probably work within three hundred miles of you in Britain. Alternatively, being not sufficiently serious about something to keep you in the UK. One pioneer's declared motive was to stay on afterwards and walk the perimeter of the island by the coast. Many others intended to tour Canada. One thing soon became clear – that few people had come because they had any opinion, for or against, those that were offered from the platform. So questions and comments amounted to zero; my anxieties were misplaced and I escaped unscathed, having nevertheless successfully influenced the world's pool of knowledge, dramatically and irreversibly.

The flight from St. John's to Montreal was passing fairly uneventfully on the way back when I was approached by a male flight attendant.

"Dr. Sagar?" he asked.

Could this be the beginnings of International fame, recognition of my revolutionary scientific discoveries, spreading already from St. John's conference hall to seat A23, Delta airlines flight D415?

"Yes," I replied, waiting for the accolade.

"Are you a doctor of medicine?"

At this point, I was tempted to embark on a discourse explaining that, in the UK at least, most "doctors" were not doctors at all but had degrees of Bachelor of Medicine and Bachelor of Surgery. Some, however, were "real" doctors because they had research degrees such as Doctor of Philosophy or indeed Doctor of Medicine. But I thought it easier, and possibly less portentous, just to say "Yes".

"Yes'" I said.

"Well, one of our female staff has a severe headache. Is that something that you could deal with?"

Sounds neurological to me, I thought. One of my friends later suggested that I had asked, "Is she pretty? If so, here I come!" but that's a bit unfair. It did lead me to wonder though whether the normal etiquette and moral rules of doctor-patient relationship applied to a passenger-flight-attendant relationship. Pure fantasy though, because even if I had been prepared to chance my arm and the General Medical Council's wrath, I doubt that she would have reciprocated because she had a headache.

I decided she probably had migraine; there was nothing urgent but she should see a(nother) neurologist with a view to further tests, including a brain scan, when on terra firma. The profundity of this advice reminded of another neurologist, Simon Coxon, who was senior registrar around the time that CAT brain scans first flourished. He was known as "CATscan Coxon" because his usual response on seeing a new referral was "I don't know the diagnosis but I am sure he/she needs a CAT scan".

The cabin crew rewarded me for my efforts with a bottle of champagne. By the way, she was pretty.

We landed and I made my way through Montreal Airport for the last leg of my return journey. After passing through Immigration, I would be on a Delta flight to Boston.

Or not. Have you ever noticed how, when things should go smoothly, they don't and, when you expect difficulties, they don't transpire? Well, this was one of the former situations.

The requirements for a non-national medic to work in the USA include not only the VQE and English test but also a work permit. Since I was in receipt of offer of work, I was granted a permit but only for six weeks initially, pending the results of the VQE and English test. When I left for Newfoundland, the results were not back so I had not received extension of the work permit and the six-week grace period had lapsed. I had realised that before I left but had an I-94 card in my passport that proved I had come from Boston and simply wanted to go back. However, a Delta official had removed the I-94 as I left the US, as is customary on leaving the country, with the assurance that it would not affect my return. Apparently, this requirement does not apply to visits to Canada of less than thirty days; if so, Mr. Delta Official was arguably a touch overzealous.

I approached the Immigration desk. I think American immigration officers are much more pleasant now (or I am less afraid of them) but at that time the expression of the lady official and the way she looked me up and down made me feel like a criminal before I had handed over any papers. She examined my passport.

"I am afraid I have to refuse you entry, sir," she said. "You do not have current valid documents."

"You are joking!" I said. On the whole, one is ill advised to use this sort of phrase when reasoning with an immigration officer but it was entirely involuntary, ma'am.

"No sir, I am not joking."

She went on to explain the nature of my problem in great detail, as if talking to an imbecile, and, as I continued profusely to object, quite how I was descending at high speed into the depths of the criminal fraternity that the USA can do without. When I got to the argument as to how the USA would lose out by not having my services, specifically because I was scheduled to do a clinic at Mass General the following morning, Boss Man came to my rescue.

"If you want somebody to help you, sir, I suggest you calm down." I felt that was an offer I could not refuse so I did.

Boss Man informed me that he had been listening in to our "conversation" (that is a euphemism, if ever I heard one) and wanted to help. He offered to telephone the Head of Immigration in Boston to check on my credentials and set off so to do. While he was away, Mrs. Grouch and I stared silently at each other in a scene reminiscent of a wild-western gun dual except that I, unlike her, was unarmed. Twenty minutes later, Boss Man returned and gave me the all-clear to board the plane.

"But I have missed the flight," I said.

"No, you haven't," said a second Delta official, to my right. "I authorise departure and I am not going to do so until this is sorted. Please, sir, now board the plane."

I got on the plane and walked to my seat with a spring in my step and, in my mind, incredulity at my good fortune. My joy was not even dampened by the other passengers, whose glowering looks alternated between me and their watch. "Who exactly is this guy for whom we all have to wait?" was at that time the single universal preoccupation of every passenger on that plane.

As I laid back in my seat and reflected on the morning, the improbability of the sequence of events slowly dawned – how easily Mr. Boss Man had located Mr. Boston Head of Immigration and how organised was the system for Mr. Boston Head of Immigration to locate my papers so quickly.

And all on a Sunday morning. No, I don't think so. Mr. Boss Man had guessed that I was an OK guy, bent the rules and applied a bit of rough justice and I was grateful. Mr. Delta Man had been pretty remarkable too.

On 17 March 1983, I wandered as usual on a Thursday morning into the office of Kath, Will's secretary, to find her clad from head to foot in green, a remarkable sight since she almost always wore grey.

"Wow, that's unusual. You look great," I said. "What's the special occasion?"

"St. Patrick's Day."

There are about thirty-six million Irish amongst the current US population of just over three hundred million. I have heard that the Irish is the largish ethnic group in the USA after the Germans, an observation that I find fascinating not because there are fewer Irish but because there are more Germans. I have been to the USA on probably a few trillion occasions to date and I don't recall seeing one German. Perhaps they all live somewhere not on my route. Many years ago, the New Yorker magazine published the New Englander's map of the USA, which consisted of an Eastern two-fifths, comprising New England, and a Western two-fifths, comprising California. Nothing else mattered. I confess that my involvement with the US has conformed to a large extent to that map where the "square states in the middle", as one Bostonian put it to me, are forgotten. Maybe the Germans live there. However, I do not want to be stereotypical, especially if I am likely to be arrested for some racist crime, so I have to admit it may equally be that our paths in New England and California have simply not crossed. Anyway, a large proportion of the Irish seemed to live in Boston.

There are about forty-five Irish pubs in Boston City itself (metro-Boston) and many more in greater Boston. If twelve percent of the US population consider themselves to be of Irish origin, as reported in one survey, and the population of metro-Boston is about six hundred thousand, about seventy-two thousand of those will be Irish, without taking account of the greater concentration of the Irish in Boston than elsewhere. A dedicated Irish-American monthly newspaper, the Boston Irish Reporter, was founded in 1990. The fact that over twenty American presidents claim to have been of Irish extraction may not be due so much to some form of Irish gerrymandering, as has been suggested, but more to there being a lot of Irish.

My father was totally Irish, and so I went to Ireland once. I found it to be very much like New York, for it was a beautiful country, and both the women and men were good-looking. James Cagney

The sense of identity is great and support for the patron saint of Ireland, St. Patrick, strong.

"Isn't the colour originally associated with St. Patrick blue?" I teased Kath.

"No, it's green."

"I think originally it was blue", I insisted (which, by the way, it was).

"Well, it's sure green now."

Kath was a stalwart old sister who could give as good as she got. We enjoyed a good banter.

"Anyway, you wouldn't understand," she sneered.

"Why not?"

"Because you're English."

"What's your Irish connection?" I asked.

"My great-grandmother was Irish," she said proudly.

"Oh, interesting, so was my grandmother," I replied.

The greater concentration of Irish genes in me compared with her was not lost on her. She went quiet, forsaking this battle so as to preserve energy for the next, which I knew she would win at all costs. By the way, Kath was short for Kathleen, which is an Irish name if ever I heard one.

We have always found the Irish a bit odd. They refuse to be English. Winston Churchill

The Irish Northern Aid Committee (NORAID) was founded in 1969 as an Irish-American fundraising organisation to promote Irish unity. Support was declared to be through peaceful means. The group came to prominence around the time that I was in Boston where many of its members were concentrated. By then, NORAID was widely suspected as being the front for the Provisional Irish Republican Army and heavily involved in raising money for arms. The US Department of Justice won a court case in 1981 forcing NORAID to register the Provisional IRA as its foreign principal but NORAID succeeded in being allowed to include a disclaimer against the ruling. Rightly or wrongly, the Irish-Americans and Boston-Irish in particular became identified as IRA sympathisers and haters of the British.

One day, Rick suggested we go into Boston for a few drinks and thought I might enjoy the Purple Shamrock in Faneuil Hall.

"With my accent?" I said. "I don't think so."

I think NORAID's current affairs had passed him by.

We finally opted for the MIT bar, where we shared a bucket of beer and a couple of reubens, which, to the uninitiated, are a disgusting variant of a hot corned beef and cheese sandwich. I had asked Rick to order something typically American for us to eat, imagining something on the grilled steak theme – or even fresh beefburger – but perhaps Rick had deliberately decided to show me how the other half eat – the half, I guess, that don't eat food.

We discussed plans for the forthcoming New York trip. One of the MIT research programmes was to test people who had had penetrating brain injuries. These folk were useful from a neuropsychological standpoint because the penetrating object, often a bullet, rather conveniently mangled just one part of the brain, leaving the others intact, and so allowed study of the intellectual functions that went missing along with that bit of brain. These injuries were quite different from closed head injuries, as sustained when the whole head collides at high speed with some unyielding object, such as a brick wall, and the brain, which has the consistency of jelly at body temperature, keeps moving within the skull. As the brain hits its own resonant frequency, to a greater or lesser extent it enters the process of global meltdown.

Part of the research examined the effects of age on brain injury so it was necessary to test these guys once each year. Since they almost all lived in New York, and like most New Yorkers were reluctant – or, in their case, unable – to leave New York, MIT staff travelled to them. The entire annual testing programme usually occupied one week.

I had been given the opportunity to go with Marie. The usual venue was no longer available so the first task was to find somewhere to stay that was cheap but had the facilities to carry out the testing. Unfortunately, the two requirements were a mutual contradiction because any hotel that had a spare room quiet enough for the subjects to concentrate on tests almost by definition fell into the "superior" category and the only place to test in a cheap hotel was in the bedroom.

After the reubenfest, I rang one hotel on the west side and suggested the latter arrangement. I indicated that a lady neuropsychologist and I would be dealing with a series of men, who would be occupied in one of our bedrooms, one at a time, for an hour or so each. For some reason, this proposal met with the news that theirs was not that kind of hotel. My first reaction was to enquire what sort of hotel specialised in the neuropsychological investigation of penetrating brain injury but I think the listener only caught the word "penetrating" and audibly began a major apoplectic fit just before putting the phone down – or hanging up, as they say over there.

Rick pointed out how someone with a deliberately depraved turn of mind could, albeit with some difficulty perhaps, misinterpret what I said so we tried an approach carefully vetted for unintended double-entendres. Eventually we found a small hotel somewhere off West 32nd Street whose proprietors agreed to our arrangements without question. After our visit to the hotel a few weeks later, I realised that they probably didn't care one iota what we did and it may well, in fact, have been precisely That Sort of Hotel.

The guys all turned up, without exception, which is quite saying something, bearing in mind that they, in toto, comprised a walking mixture of memory, judgement and planning deficits. Maybe reliability on such occasions is an American characteristic because I also noticed that the patients at the Mass General clinics also tended to turn up - certainly more often than NHS patients in England, anyway. You could argue that the American patients attended seemingly conscientiously because they were paying for the service – it's easier to ignore something that is being given free – but, in truth, most of them had private health insurance and would not personally pay anything. However, the New York brain-injured had little to gain by turning up, except perhaps the comfort that someone at least was interested in their plight.

Jake Wheeler was one of the most brain damaged such that he could not make his own way to the hotel and had to be brought by his brother. Jake was another patient with frontal lobe injury. In his case, however, it had produced a pattern of thinking similar to schizophrenia. He would seemingly answer a question satisfactorily but careful examination showed that his responses, although apparently direct, were in fact tangential but barely enough to notice. "One step forward and one to the side" or "the knight's move in conversation" (after the movement pattern of the chess piece) are often used to describe this pattern of conversation. It was easy to be drawn progressively, albeit without deliberate intention on his part, away from the subject of the conversation. Attempts to keep on track were very wearing. As a psychiatrist once said, "If after talking for thirty minutes, you do not know whether it is them who is mad or you, the diagnosis is schizophrenia." Harsh, perhaps, but with a ring of truth for Jake who had a similar disorder of thinking. After half an hour with him, I felt exhausted and not quite sane.

A coffee break at the local diner was essential.

We joined the line at the counter and reached the attendant at the end in no time because time is one thing that New Yorkers do not have.

"Yes?" she snapped at Rick.

"Cappuccino," he responded quickly.

"You?" Her question was accompanied by a finger pointed, with uncanny accuracy, towards the region of my heart.

"Erm ...," I began.

"Two cappuccinos," she shouted to the bank of coffee-making men and women lined in front of a steaming steel machine to her rear. Clearly fifty microseconds was the maximum time allowed by US Federal Law to answer the question.

We sat down at one of the twenty tables, all closely cramped together. To my left, was a couple with opposing accents: his was Bronx New York; hers was cut-crystal English. What were they doing together, I wondered, but they seemed to be an item of one kind or another.

A waitress, marginally less aggressive than the lady who had previously helped me, strode over to their table.

"What can I get you?" she asked.

"Cheeseburger, fries and regular coke," he said with no hesitation.

"You?" she nodded to the girl.

"Please may I have a small Caesar salad and a glass of tap water?" she said, in impeccable English but faulty American.

"What'd she say?" she snapped at the man.

"Small Caesar, regular water," he punched back at her.

"Sure." She turned on her heel and was gone almost before she said the word.

After their meal, a smiling third female employee sauntered over with the bill. It seemed as if the staff became logarithmically slower the longer we stayed in the restaurant.

No doubt some variant of Einstein's Theory of Relativity could explain it.

Having received payment, by credit card of course, she said to the couple.

"Thank you. Have a nice day here in New York."

The English girl, keen in the pursuit of clarity, said, "Actually, we are here for two weeks."

"Well, have a nice day while you are here," said the waitress. "Which one?" I felt like asking but refrained.

Refreshed by the fortuitous entertainment rather more than the coffee, we returned to the state-of-the-art cognitive-testing lab at Hotel That-Kind-Of to resume work at the front line of science. Each day for the rest of the week, we returned to the same diner to see whether any of the personalities, working conditions and staff-customer banter had changed. They hadn't.

End of week. Job done. Back to Boston and relative peace.

A stay in the USA should be at least two years, the second year being to confirm the veracity of the observations of the first year: the seasons, the food, the weather, the countryside, the bugs. Novel experiences following each other in rapid succession was like a second childhood although not in the sense that might be applied to some of my Alzheimer patients.

The seasons: someone living in Britain would be forgiven for not knowing the season, even if their mental capacity was intact, because each one has components of the others (even winter in spring/summer – for example, snow fell in Sheffield on 2 June 1975 causing disruption of a Derbyshire versus Lancashire cricket match at Buxton when an inch of snow fell on the pitch, a local disaster). In the USA, or Massachusetts at least, the season leaves you in no doubt. The official climate statistics for Boston suggest a relatively gradual transition between the seasons. In my experience, however, spring doesn't exist. When I was there, the temperature hovered around fifty degrees Fahrenheit for weeks until Memorial Day, the last Monday in May, when it rose by about thirty degrees overnight and stayed there. The rhododendrons all came into bloom simultaneously and wilted en masse about two days later.

Somebody somewhere just managed to fit a season between summer and winter, probably because, without it, the spectacle of the New England fall with landscapes of trees in bright red, orange and yellow would not exist. And the Bostonians would not be able to vacate the city in their hundreds for one of the "inns" in Vermont to gaze at the trees. So popular was this habit that inn bookings were made preferably before birth in order to guarantee a reservation during one's lifetime. Anyway, it would probably take that long to accumulate the necessary resources to pay for the accommodation unless, of course, you were prepared to stay for less than one night. (Dear Mister US Ambassador, the last two sentences are not really quite true. The inns are great and the trees are beautiful. You have designed both very well.)

The food: food is important to Americans, except those with anorexia, of whom there are not many. Most of the food is good. OK, so the Italians invented pizza; the Germans invented hamburgers and hotdogs, or at least frankfurters; and Coca Cola began as Pemberton's French Wine Cola based on vin mariana, a coca wine from Bordeaux - but the Americans do it all better – or at least, differently and well. It's also worth noting that, without America, Europe would not have a pizza tomato sauce because the tomato probably began its life in Peru. Although strictly speaking Peru is in South America, the USA can arguably still claim more credit because New York, a mainstay of pizza consumption, is closer to Peru at around three thousand six hundred miles than is Italy at around six thousand seven hundred miles.

The Americans have thus managed to harvest talent from overseas and exploited it. According to the BBC, even ice cream was imported from China via Arabia and Europe but the US clearly latched on quickly because it was already being served by George Washington, the first President of the USA, and the first ice cream parlour opened in New York City as early as 1776. Maybe the USA would never have been formed without ice cream.

By the time of my arrival, ice cream evolution had led to ice cream chocolates, made with fresh cream, at Legal Seafoods in Kendall Square, a regular haunt of the MIT Psychology Department, not least because it was about five minutes away on foot. Closer to our US home was Kimball's Farm, at Westford, eight miles north of Acton, which served the best ice cream I have ever tasted. Judging by current subscribers to tripadvisor.com, I was not and am still not alone. Portions were huge but the Kimball's Special surpassed all. For a few dollars, you could be the proud recipient of the equivalent of a large tureen piled to a depth of about two feet at the centre with a mixture of Kimball's richest flavours. It was wise to avoid food for a few weeks before embarking on a Kimball's Special Challenge. Even then, very few people managed to complete it, as witnessed by the contents of large waste bins, swarming with flies, across the road from the serving hatch.

The bugs: in keeping with the general observation that the USA has more of everything from food to weather, it also has more bugs (certainly more than Europe; I doubt that my generalisation applies to the Amazon rainforest and possibly not subsaharan Africa either but, either way, enough is enough).

One day, around mid-June of the first year, we were sitting in our apartment when, seemingly within a few minutes, the double French windows leading to the garden became covered with a mass of fifteen-millimetre-diameter brown objects. The effect on light transmission into the apartment was not far removed from that of a total eclipse of the sun. The initial conclusion that we were recipients of a large deposit of nuclear dust courtesy of the USSR (the Soviet bloc did not begin to collapse until 1989) was dispelled when we realised that the brown bodies had independent motion skills in the form of six legs each. Welcome to Popillia japonica, the Japanese beetle. This little beauty comes out to play around June and July after a year in development and, before embarking on its main task in life of generating yet more Popillia, seeks to destroy by consumption every plant it fancies, which is most of them.

The United States Department of Agriculture (USDA) Animal Plant Health Inspection Service in its Program Aid 1599, issued in July 1977 and revised April 2004, informs us that the USDA "prohibits discrimination in all its programmes and activities on the basis of race, colour, national origin, sex, religion, age, disability, political beliefs, sexual orientation or marital or family status". Obviously this doesn't apply to Popillia japonica whose "national origin" is Japan because the USDA regards it as "a highly destructive plant pest of foreign origin" and "a threat to American agriculture". Hence the USDA has a list of recommendations to limit the problem, including a number of chemicals useful for destruction of both young and adult forms of the Japanese immigrant.

Unfortunately, the conclusion of Program Aid 1599 is that the recommended program "will not eliminate all Japanese beetles from your property". I am able to confirm that, without any such control measures, and quite possibly with them also, Poppy and his extended family make a very similar pattern of return every twelve months. Fortunately they don't hang around long, are surprisingly quite attractive and are little trouble as long as you are not a plant.

Not so the greenhead fly (Tabanus nigrovittatus). If you are ever tempted to escape the Japanese beetle by holidaying on Plum Island, Massachusetts, don't, at least if it's July 1983. Tabanus nigrovittatus sets up camp there from June to September and is not fond of visitors. Consequently, a walk through the dunes becomes an exercise in self-preservation worthy of the Special Boat Squadron as hundreds of the horsefly variant descend on bodies and hair, determined to bite the victims into either departure or extinction. The only way to get by is to swing any available piece of clothing in a constant rotatory fashion around the head, like a helicopter, to prevent their landing. Apart from the near drowning of my daughter, which, to be fair, had nothing to do with Tabanus, the greenheaders made our first visit to Plum Island quite memorable. For our second trip, we selected different delights by avoiding June to September and preventing my daughter from testing out the fierce undercurrents of the shore using a bucket so large she could hardly lift it.

I understand that the greenhead fly has, in recent years, been subject to severe population control so the hazard is nowhere near so great. Mental note: must go back one July.

The one six-legged friend we managed to avoid was the cockroach – except once when I saw one crawling across the bedroom floor. To the credit of the letting agency, he and any of his accompanying friends were sent to cockroach heaven within twenty-four hours by mass fumigation. The experience was doubtless better than that of our friends in Arizona who befriended black widow spiders and tarantulas in their garden for one month at a time until the regular fumigation service turfed them out motionless on their backs.

By the time of our planned return to the UK, we had somehow gained a six-week-old baby boy. We thought we had better check on his nationality before departure and so phoned the US Immigration Department:

"We are a British couple who gave birth to a son in Boston six weeks ago. What nationality is he?"

"American," came the immediate and brusk reply.

We then phoned the British Embassy:

"We are a British couple who gave birth to a son in Boston six weeks ago. What nationality is he?"

"Why, British, of course," she said with a smile in her voice.

And so his dual nationality was born. When it came to passports, the American one had to carry a photograph of the boy. The one we included bore a startling resemblance to him but also to every other six-week-old child in the world.

We thought that the Yank-Brit hybrid would have fitted for the journey into one of the suitcases but the airline thought it generally better to provide a cot for the flight. That seemed to take care of one half of the progeny. After six hours or so of entertaining the other, we touched down at Heathrow.

In America there are two classes of travel - first class, and with children. Robert Benchley

Chapter 8:   Fruition

Fresh fruit can be preserved or left to be consumed, rot or turn to alcohol.

Mine was a new post, increasing to four the consultant contingent in neurology. The catchment population for the Department of Neurology was around 2.3 million, giving us nearly six hundred thousand potential patients each. Perhaps it's not surprising that the waiting lists were long. By comparison, virtually the same population in 2013 is served by about twenty consultants. It is difficult to be more precise about the number because most people are not sure who the consultants are.

The plan of clinical work was fairly established by twelve months into the job: inpatients, ward rounds, outpatient clinics and ward referrals. I had an office to myself, having successfully relocated my secretary who had shared my office until then. Not only were we fed up with being in each other's company but she seemed to be a little inhibited in her more intimate telephone calls in my presence. Most importantly, my colleagues had heard enough moaning from me about not having an office on my own. My specialist clinic in movement disorders, particularly Parkinson's disease, was now in full flight.

In 1984, all clinics, with one exception, were held in Sheffield and all four consultants did regular weekly clinics and ward rounds. In 2012, clinics are carried out regularly at other hospitals in the region so consultants are often not present in the teaching hospital. Moreover, not all are engaged in full clinical duties at the same time.

The exception to the universal siting of clinics in Sheffield was one day each week spent by me in Doncaster, approximately twenty miles from Sheffield. Doncaster's main claim to fame, before the arrival of neurology, was transport. The town's website informs us that the stagecoach trade of the seventeenth and eighteenth centuries generated the wealth that built the Georgian town centre and horse breeding for the trade gave rise to the Doncaster racecourse.   Apparently, Doncaster's strong standing in the railway industry included amazing engineering works that built the Flying Scotsman locomotive amongst others. More recently, Doncaster and its surrounding area was a thriving base for the coal industry. Apart from the racecourse, none of this was terribly obvious when viewed from the route to Doncaster Royal Infirmary, which is a pleasant enough but not exciting building built in stages between 1930 and 1989 and paying little compliment to the Georgian town centre (which is itself not obvious).

The Doncaster day soon established a pattern: morning clinic and afternoon ward referrals, followed by domiciliary visits in late afternoon and evening. The clinics usually comprised, to varying degrees, a neurological pick-and-mix of headaches, dizzy spells, blackouts, numb bits, sensitive bits, numb and sensitive bits, shakes, rattles, rolls and most other things that you can imagine. Neurology is a speciality dealing with problems affecting the brain and nervous system which work by electrical conduction. So a neurologist is essentially an electrician as a cardiologist is a plumber and a plastic surgeon a painter and decorator. When someone develops a wiring fault, something, dependent on that wiring, fails. Since most bodily functions are controlled by nerves, the possible results of neurological failure are serious and widespread. It is arguments like that that persuade neurologists that they are important.

"Hello, Mr. Turner, what seems to be the problem?"

"I was hoping you were going to tell me that," he replied unthreateningly, with a half-smile on his face. The Doncaster clinic had begun in typical fashion.

"Well, what have you noticed?"

"Nothing," he said. "If anything's the problem, that's it."

"Why?"

"Because my family thinks there is a problem. They told me to come."

"Have they come with you?" I asked, more in hope than expectation.

"No." The predictable answer.

"What have they told you is wrong?" I knew that, if the answer to this was also "Nothing", we had no history, no symptoms, no complaint. Making a diagnosis in a state of total communication blackout can be a little tricky. Fortunately, some information was forthcoming.

"They say I have funny turns."

"Can you tell me what they have noticed?"

"They say that I suddenly stop speaking and just stare straight ahead. After a while, I come round and act as if nothing has happened."

"After how long?"

"Not sure but from what they said it sounds like less than a minute, I would think."

Attacks like that are often minor seizures, a form of epilepsy. Usually, but not always, the patients will also have more severe attacks, such as the major convulsion that most people understand by an epileptic fit. I was concerned because Mr. Turner was aged sixty-two; epilepsy developing at that age is more likely to be due to something serious, such as a brain tumour, than epilepsy starting earlier in life.

"Have you ever had a more severe attack, such as one where you collapse on the floor?"

"No."

"How long have you had these dos?" I asked.

"About forty years."

"Forty years!" Even I, with twelve or more years under my belt as a doctor, was surprised.

"Have you never been to the doctor about them?"

"No, because I have never felt anything wrong. I have certainly never felt ill with them."

"So why come now?"

"My granddaughter made me come. I think she is worried about me. I didn't want to upset her so I said I would come."

"But your wife and children have known about these dos?"

"Yes, but when it happened, they just said Dad is having one of his turns."

I told him my suspicions concerning epilepsy but we agreed that, since he had had the attacks for so long and nothing worse had developed, and he had no intention of taking medication even if some doctor were daft enough to suggest it, nothing more would be done. Sadly, Mr. Turner came to please his granddaughter and gained nothing except the news that the attacks rendered him ineligible to drive and he must inform the licensing authority. Whether he did so is, of course, quite another matter.

Three weeks after that, I was asked to see a twenty-nine-year-old lady on the ward. She had been admitted as an emergency with two major epileptic seizures over the course of twelve hours with no relevant past history. She had fully recovered by the time I saw her and neurological examination revealed no abnormality. She wanted to go home. However, I recommended a brain scan because I was concerned at the occurrence of two seizures in rapid succession for no obvious reason. Later that day, her consultant telephoned me to say that the scan showed multiple deposits of cancer throughout the brain. It didn't take long to discover that the primary source of the cancer was a malignant melanoma, a nasty form of skin cancer. It didn't take long because, six weeks later, we had what is sometimes referred to as "the benefit of a post-mortem" (quite who benefits is difficult to say). She had died in another seizure.

It is rarely sufficient in neurology to make a diagnosis of epilepsy or stroke or multiple sclerosis or indeed most conditions because each one has a range of severity from mild and of no dire consequence to severe, incapacitating and possibly life-threatening. A powerful argument is that a diagnosis has little importance in its own right; what is important is what is going to be done in a certain medical situation and what will happen in the future. The diagnosis is important only as a guide to these principles. However, that does not stop doctors being obsessed with them.

Each Thursday afternoon, I would while away the hours on happy excursions around the medical, surgical and orthopaedic wards, reviewing patients at their consultant's request. These "ward referrals" were ostensibly and indeed usually genuinely made to seek advice on the diagnosis or management of a patient with a neurological disorder. However, all consultants, including myself, sometimes confer with a colleague because they haven't a clue what is going on with their patient and wonder if the cause may be neurological/cardiological/psychiatric or, in fact, any speciality other than their own. It is here that the obsessive diagnostician comes into his or her own because, not having the overall responsibility for the patient, they can limit their confidence to the boundary of their diagnostic comfort zone.

"Thank you for asking me to see this patient. I do not think the diagnosis is multiple sclerosis, as you have asked, because the lesions on the brain scans are not typical and the onset of MS is unusual at this patient's age. Moreover, I felt there was poor cooperation from the patient in the testing of power in the lower limbs so the apparent weakness is probably not genuine."

Here endeth the epistle. The skill in the generation of these entries in the patient's notes is to raise more questions than are answered and to imply, without actually stating, that at least part of the problem is the fault of the patient, either because of deliberate misrepresentation or because they are barking mad.

The thoughts of the author of this entry in the patient's notes are quite different from the written version:

"I wish you hadn't asked me to see this patient because I do not know what is wrong with them. Unfortunately, I can't easily get out of the situation because the brain scan is abnormal so they have obviously got a neurological disorder and you have asked the appropriate specialist. I can tell you what the diagnosis is not, which may get me off the hook, at least temporarily. If I can find any evidence that may implicate another speciality as well as my own, I can procrastinate until the responsible consultant has conferred with the other specialist and argued on the relative contribution of neurology and this other speciality. That will give me time to look at the books and reflect a while. We all know that a psychological disorder is difficult to prove or disprove because there are no relevant tests so I will suggest that. And anyway, I don't think that <u>all</u> of the weakness is genuine so that much is true."

Some consultants nurture this mode of thinking into a positive art form. You will see it most often in situations where its practitioner can sound off without major consequence, such as at research conferences and in courts of law where it will not be a life-or-death issue whether or not their opinion is heeded (and where it is difficult to prove that they are wrong). As in the example above, the key component of the art is to offer no opinion at all on the actual diagnosis and to confine one's comments to what is not wrong or to imply that the suggested diagnosis is a startling irrelevance.

As heard in a court of law:

"Do you agree that this patient has MS?"

"No, because the presentation is not typical."

"So what is the cause of the abnormal brain scan, which presumably shows why the patient cannot walk?"

"Even if the diagnosis is MS, I do not believe that it is responsible for the walking difficulty."

And this:

"Do you agree that this lady has the diagnosis of dopa-responsive dystonia?"

"No."

"Why not?"

"Because she is the wrong age. All the patients in the series of dopa-responsive dystonia described by Segawa were children or adolescents. This lady is aged twenty-two. Her condition is beyond the pale."

"But do you agree she has dystonia?"

"Yes."

"And do you agree that it is responsive to dopa?"

"Yes."

"So she has dopa-responsive dystonia?"

"She doesn't have the *diagnosis* of dopa-responsive dystonia."

"What does she have then?"

"I don't know."

Or this heard at a research conference:

"Dr. Westcott, do you agree that lamotrigine is effective treatment for migraine?"

"Yes, the CALM study – that is Carbamazepine And Lamotrigine in Migraine – showed that lamotrigine was superior to placebo in reducing the frequency and severity of migraine attacks."

"What is the best dose?"

"The dose in that study was six hundred milligrams daily."

"Is that the best dose? I ask because I find four hundred milligrams daily to be just as effective with fewer side effects."

"Don't know. Haven't done the trials."

"What's your impression?"

"I am afraid we haven't done the trials."

A peculiar thing in medicine is that we never believe anything unless it can be demonstrated in animals. John A. Schindler, M.D.

At least Dr. Westcott was being honest but sometimes ill patients are not prepared to wait until the research has been done before someone attempts to make them better. And aspirin was used for treatment of pain, digitalis for heart failure and phenobarbitone for epilepsy long before a clinical trial was even a glimmer in its father's eye. Fortunately, most of the time, we do not have to engage in these diversionary discussions because often the diagnosis and treatment would be obvious to a half-trained primate. A doctor's skill is more concerned with meaningful interaction with a patient as an individual than simple recognition and treatment of a medical disorder in an abstract sense.

So many come to the sickroom thinking of themselves as men of science fighting disease and not as healers with a little knowledge helping nature to get a sick man well. Auckland Geddes "The Practitioner"

One day, I was called to the medical ward by Dr. Hickens, a consultant physician, to see a middle-aged lady who had had episodes of loss of vision with mild headache. After the usual introductions, I asked her about her attacks.

"The vision in my right eye goes suddenly. My husband says it's a blackout."

"Well, in one sense, I suppose it is, but ...."

"So you agree with him then?"

"Well, the term blackout can cover a multitude of problems. Certainly, it sounds as if your vision blacks out."

"My obstetrician says my vision is fine."

"Your obstetrician?"

"The man who checked my eyes."

"Oh, your optician, yes I see."

"My doctor says its My Grain," she said, with equal stress on the "My" and "Grain" and a staccato-like separation between the two words.

"Migraine, yes possibly."

After learning of several more diagnoses volunteered to Mrs. Johnson by members of various professions and the lay public, I was able to pin her down long enough to be able to extract some relevant information.

"Are there any conditions that run in your family?" I asked.

"Well, my father had trouble with his preposterous gland. He couldn't pass water."

"Prostate gland, yes."

"Yes, prostrate gland."

"And my cousin had celeriac disease. He couldn't eat wheat and had to have a glutinous free diet."

"Thank you. Coeliac disease treated with a gluten-free diet. Yes. Anything else?"

"My uncle had a problem with his gall bladder. He couldn't pass water either."

"Sorry, Mrs. Johnson," I said, "there is the bladder, sometimes called the urinary bladder, which we use to pass water. The gall bladder is different; it lies near the stomach. It sounds as if the problem was with his ordinary or urinary bladder."

"Well, he also had indigestion."

"Anything else?"

"My mother had a gastric stomach."

After thirty to forty minutes, I felt like a United Nations linguist carrying out translations of speeches in real time but had gleaned enough to conclude what was wrong with her. I explained:

"The problem is that, from time to time, the blood supply to your eye becomes blocked. Without its blood supply, the eye cannot function so you lose your vision. However, after a short time, the blockage opens up; the blood supply returns to your eye and your vision comes back."

"I think that's what Dr. Hickens thought. He said it might be a transit anaemic attack."

"It's actually called a transient ischaemic attack," I said, "transient meaning temporary and ischaemic loss of blood supply. So its an attack consisting of a temporary loss of blood supply."

"Why am I having transit anaemic attacks?" she asked.

"Well, we need to find out. We will have to do some tests to look at the circulation."

"Ah, circular problems run in the family too. My aunt had vigorous veins."

"Well, varicose veins are actually a bit different."

"So it's not My Grain?"

"Well, it could be migraine but I think it is important to make sure that there isn't a problem with your arteries."

"So the tests will look at my hearties?"

"Yes."

Varicose veins are the result of an improper selection of grandparents. William Osler

We transferred her to Sheffield for an angiogram, an X-ray of the arteries to the brain. My registrar wrote to her after her discharge from hospital to confirm the results. He was not a great communicator. His letter started off well: "Dear Mrs. Johnson, I am writing to let you know the result of the X-ray of the blood vessels in your neck."

So far, so good. But then: "This shows extensive atheroma extending from the carotid bifurcation to the Circle of Willis bilaterally. As discussed when you were an inpatient, such lesions are not amenable to surgery."

I hate to think what Mrs. Johnson made of that when recounting the findings to others.

For a doctor, modern medicine is a strange hybrid of science and clinical skills, which live uncomfortably together like a married couple who don't get on but cannot do without each other. Science, of course, leads to medical advances and, by its very nature, is precise. Clinical skills represent more of an art form taking simultaneously into account the history of someone who is in no position to know the relative significance of one symptom over another, vague or non-existent signs on physical examination and a host of intuitary skills, assessing mode of presentation and body language of the patient. A doctor needs to assess the significance of what is unsaid as well as what is said.

In the sick room, ten cents' worth of human understanding equals ten dollars' worth of medical science. Martin H. Fischer

The arch proponents of scientific or "evidence-based medicine" as it is known in the trade would probably represent the right wing if medicine were transformed into politics, whilst the poor clinician, battling with soft policies, an uphill battle to get people better and a holistic approach to the patient as a person and not simply a vehicle for disease, would be firmly on the left. As we have seen, the right-winger can confine himself to situations for which there is a good scientific approach whilst not concerning himself with the witch-doctor methods of his softer colleagues. Some would argue that, with sufficient scientific advance, and consequent knowledge of the workings and failings of the human body, medicine could conquer all aliments and all disease, disorder and bodily malfunction would disappear forever. Others are religious.

What happens then is like what happens when we separate a jigsaw puzzle into its five hundred pieces: The over-all picture disappears. This is the state of modern medicine: It has lost the sense of the unity of man. Such is the price it has paid for its scientific progress. It has sacrificed art to science. Paul Tournier, M.D.

It is true that disease can be conquered. For probably a few thousand years, smallpox had ruled the roost through most of the world, wiping out anyone it didn't fancy and disabling many more. Its authority had overruled King Louis XV of France, Tsar Peter II of Russia and Queen Mary II of England by removing them from their thrones and sending them underground. It has been said that smallpox killed one child in ten in Sweden and France and one in seven in Russia even by the eighteenth century. Survivors were facially disfigured from deep scars, known as pockmarks, often blind and decidedly unattractive.

Milkmaids, by contrast, often had unblemished faces and good vision and were pretty, at least relatively so. The farming community had reportedly long recognised that infection with cowpox from cows' udders produced only a mild, non-disabling disease but provided protection from the much nastier smallpox. By the late eighteenth century, the widespread knowledge of the rural population had finally filtered down to the medical profession, at least that proportion that lived in towns. Dr. Fewster from Thornbury, Gloucestershire, presented a paper to the Medical Society of London in 1765 entitled "Cowpox and its ability to prevent smallpox". These observations prompted Edward Jenner to test deliberately the effect of the administration of cowpox on the later risk of acquisition of smallpox.

A milkmaid, Sarah Nelmes, went to see Edward Jenner for treatment of cowpox. Doctor Jenner extracted fluid from the cowpox pustules and injected them into James

Phipps, the eight-year-old son of his gardener. James contracted a mild case of cowpox but recovered. The physician then injected him with smallpox but James showed no reaction; he was immune to smallpox. As a result of this and later experiments, Edward Jenner has been credited with founding the principle of vaccination to provide resistance against infectious diseases.

This story should come with a "Do not try this at home" warning because, these days, Mr. Phipps would be required to provide informed consent on behalf of his underage son with death from smallpox being deemed to be an acceptable outcome and the General Medical Council may have something to say about the ethics of the experiment. Fee-hungry lawyers may not have much difficulty in establishing a case of medical negligence if something went wrong either. Anyway, the good news is that these little considerations clearly did not hamper the medical entrepreneurs of the day and vaccination for smallpox was born.

By the early 1950s, approximately fifty million cases of smallpox occurred in the world each year, but increasing vaccination led to a fall to around ten to fifteen million by 1967. In that year, the World Health Organisation launched a programme of mass world-wide vaccination which led to formal recognition of the global eradication of the disease in 1980.

The last natural case was in Somalia in 1977. I always feel sorry for that person - if only the spread of the disease had stopped just one person earlier.

But that's the only human disease that has ever been eradicated. Moreover, despite official declaration by the World Health Organisation in 1980 that smallpox no longer exists as an infection of people, the USA (Centers for Disease Control and Prevention, CDC) and Russia (The State Research Center of Virology and Biotechnology VECTOR, also known as the Vector Institute) continue to stockpile the virus. The official reasons for so doing are in case smallpox comes back and for possible research into resistance against biological warfare. Quite why this is necessary if the virus doesn't exist anywhere else is unclear. Even the provision of jobs for unemployed and purposeless researchers hardly seems an overriding consideration. The need for techniques to resist smallpox warfare exists only as long as there is a possibility of using smallpox virus as an aggressive agent which exists only as long as the virus is stockpiled. So we have a wonderful self-reinforcing situation. Fortunately, potential use of the virus as an active agent of warfare is strongly denied by all authorities so it looks as if we can all rest easy in our beds.

The CDC website informs us: "The September 11, 2001 terrorist attacks in the United States raised concerns about the possible use of biological weapons such as smallpox. CDC helped prepare for such an attack by working with state and local health departments to vaccinate civilian health care response team members, so they could safely care for patients with smallpox."

"More than 44,000 people were vaccinated against smallpox as part of the National Smallpox Pre-Event Vaccination Program, launched on December 13, 2002. CDC's Immunization Safety Office (ISO) helped monitor the vaccine's safety." Oh dear! How depressing - poor old Jenner must be turning in his grave.

Before closing the subject of smallpox, I should point out that Edward Jenner was probably not the first to use cowpox vaccination against smallpox. Benjamin Jesty, a Dorset farmer, who had previously had cowpox, infected his wife Elizabeth and their two sons with cowpox in an attempt to provide resistance against smallpox when an epidemic came to Yetminster in 1774. They all recovered and did not catch smallpox.

As rewards for discovering and promoting vaccination, Edward Jenner received rewards from the House of Commons of ten thousand pounds in June 1802, and twenty thousand pounds in 1807. George Pearson, founder of the Original Vaccine Pock Institution, gave evidence of Benjamin Jesty's work of 1774, twenty-two years before Jenner's, but various factors mitigated against Jesty's well-documented case and he received nothing. I expect he's turning in his grave as well.

In science, credit goes to the man who convinces the world, not the man to whom the idea first occurs. Francis Galton

Scientific progress in medicine is not lost on patients whose access to the internet has supplanted mother's words of wisdom as the major information resource, director and comforter.

Tony Ward was referred to me by Dr. Bolton, Consultant in General Medicine, with a suspected diagnosis of peripheral neuropathy. Peripheral neuropathy is a condition in which the nerve fibres, mostly in the arms and legs, die off and cause weakness and numbness. The smallest nerve fibres are affected first and the condition then spreads to larger ones, in a pattern similar to the death of small twigs on a tree followed by involvement of larger and larger branches. As a result, symptoms of peripheral neuropathy start at the ends of the fingers and toes and spread back gradually up the limbs.

It was fairly soon apparent that the diagnosis of Mr. Ward was correct so I began to explain that peripheral neuropathy had many causes and we would need to do further tests to find out more. At this point, TW dived into his briefcase by the side of his chair and pulled out more paper than I thought the briefcase could possibly accommodate. His wife was already holding about another half ream, presumably the excess that the poor briefcase could not cope with.

"We googled peripheral neuropathy and came up with some information that you may be familiar with. However, we thought that we would bring it along for your comments," he said, possibly a touch patronisingly.

I made a quick assessment that, at fifteen minutes' discussion per page, we could be involved in discussion for about two weeks provided we limited ourselves to eight hours per day. I hastily tried to steer him back to the more traditional roles whereby I was the giver, and he the recipient, of information. But I soon began to feel like a medical student being chastised for knowing next to nothing and not even bothering to open a text book in possibly a vain attempt to correct my inadequacy.

"Nobody has checked us for diabetes," he said.

This use of the first person plural "us" and "we" came to be a recurrent component of the discussion, if that is what it could be called, as if his wife had been sucked irrevocably into the whole disease process.

"Dr. Bolton checked your blood glucose and it was normal. That effectively excludes diabetes," I said, in as reassuring a tone as I could muster.

"Effectively perhaps but not definitely because it depends when the blood test is done. If we haven't eaten anything, we can't have any glucose in our blood."

"Well, that's not quite correct Mr. Ward. In fact, we often check the blood glucose level after a period of starvation as a better test for diabetes."

"It's not better in our opinion."

He fumbled amongst his papers and I fully expected him to extract an article that he would see as the coup de grace to my authority – something like "Fasting Blood Glucose Misdiagnoses Diabetes" by I.M. Expert-Wannabee, MD (failed) in the Journal of Bad Research 1873. But he had moved on.

"What about acrylamide poisoning?" he offered. Acrylamide is a chemical used in various industrial processes and can sometimes cause a neuropathy.

"That is very rare. Have you ever worked in an industry that uses acrylamide?"

"No but it's present in food," he said, a little too emphatically perhaps.

Indeed, acrylamide is present in food, especially chips and other starchy foods, but how he knew that I don't know because that discovery was only made in 2002 and we were still in 1999. I expect he made a lucky guess but, since he was holding a sheaf of a few dozen pieces of paper when he said it, I found it difficult to be sure that the internet had not provided at least some backing for his claim.

"It will not be present in food in toxic quantities," I boldly suggested, hoping he wasn't going to break into a grin and slap an internet printout on my desk in the manner of a parent beating his child at the game, Happy Families: sympathetic but inwardly delighted at the exercise of superior intellect and control. Luckily, he didn't respond and I was safe.

The beauty of the internet for self-researchers is that indiscriminate searches will usually find some site that provides information to back any theory you care to put forward. Mr. Ward failed to find a backing for his idea that he had been rendered neurologically disabled by McDonald's fries, not because such support did not exist somewhere, however unreliably, but more likely that he had not searched hard enough.

Work at the hospital completed, the Doncaster day would typically end with a series of domiciliary visits. A rather quaint leftover from the period when consultants had some status, a domiciliary visit was a consultation with a patient in their own home at the request of the general practitioner. I cannot state with any certainty but I suspect the arrangement initially involved a certain amount of forelock-tugging and Uriah Heep impersonation on the part of the requesting general practitioner and a considered, aloof response on the part of the consultant as he reflected whether the problem described was of sufficient importance for him – and it was universally him in those days – to create a gap in his diary already overfilled with appointments of groundbreaking significance. The general practitioner was expected to be present at the domiciliary visit and may well have been required to present the history of the case to the consultant with a subservience only slightly less than that of a fledgling house officer. In truth, this could have had some benefit to the GP as he appeared to the patient exceptionally smart in arranging the services of someone so important.

The domiciliary visit was supposed to accommodate those patients who were too ill to attend an outpatient department but not sufficiently ill to be admitted to hospital – or where the GP was uncertain of the urgency of the situation. But you can bet your life that the exercise was embedded in a social framework in which the actors on the medical stage each acted out their part according to an unwritten but mutually recognised script. The interdependence between GP and consultant and acceptance by both of a certain behaviour pattern was motivated, as always, by money. If Mr. GP referred lots of domiciliary visits to Mr. Consultant, Mr. GP would bypass the outpatient department waiting list, be popular with his patients and be relieved of the stress of how to get rid of a difficult medical problem. Because a domiciliary visit attracted a fee, Mr. Consultant would meanwhile make loads of money.

By my time, all this pretence had gone. Only once, early in my consultant career, did I have the GP present at the visit and that may have been to see how attractive I was because I later discovered he was gay. (There may be a flaw in this argument because straight male GPs did not accompany female consultants on domiciliary visits either.) The GP didn't always bother even to speak to me personally; quite often, the request was via a message left with my secretary and passed on to me with varying degrees of precision. I never did quite work out why things had changed. I knew consultants still did domiciliary visits for the money so their motivation had not changed. Something must have happened to the GPs. Maybe they got fed up with sucking up to consultants or no longer felt the need for patient approval. Maybe they were too busy. Or maybe they were now paid so much they didn't care what anyone thought.

The domiciliary experience was certainly educational and not particularly from the standpoint of medical knowledge. First, I learnt so much local geography I could have pursued a second career as a satnav – if satnavs had existed then, which they didn't. Unfortunately. The patients invariably lived in some remote village in the Doncaster coalfield where the local council had insufficient funds, ability or motivation to produce street signs or perhaps where the streets had never been named at all ("street on the right past the blacksmith's shop"). Anyway, for whatever reason, my spatial orientation was not assisted by any useful visual clue. I usually had to resort to asking one – or several – locals. Usually, it was several because each one was only sufficiently certain of the localisation of Mr. X's house "even though I see him every day" to direct me to the next street en route where further enquiry was required.

The problem became more acute as night fell because not only were roads and houses harder to identify in the dark but the streets also became increasingly deserted of willing assistance. Sometimes the exodus of life from these South Yorkshire byways was so fast as to give the impression of arrival soon after some local catastrophe: children's bicycles strewn at an angle, half on the pavement, half on the road; half-eaten packet of crisps, lying on top of the privet hedge; car door ajar with internal light blazing and Tesco carrier bag on the back seat; Doberman Pinscher standing motionless on the garden path with uncharacteristic timidity and a puzzled expression. It resembled the Marie Celeste, in so far as bicycles, crisps, cars and Doberman Pinschers existed in December 1872 when the ship was found drifting crewless but unharmed in the Atlantic Ocean.

As the year progressed, I noticed that the termination of Yorkshire human life coincided with dusk only at certain times of the year; sometimes, it was before and sometimes after. Taking into account the fact that the hours of daylight varied according to the season, I was able to conclude that it was the time and not the nightfall that was the critical precipitant of the fleeing from the Doncaster coalfield. When the loss of light and life coincided, I felt particularly abandoned. I was never sure of the cause of the human evacuation but suspect it was the unlocking of the pub door, the pinging of the microwave or both, depending on age and gender.

Once the street had been located, the next goal was to find the house, a task not particularly assisted in many cases by the design of the estate. Subsections, each consisting of say twenty houses, were aligned with each other in almost random orientation such that the house number from one block did not flow seamlessly into the numbering of the next block. A journey from number twenty-five to twenty-six may involve a walk down a side road, a right turn and a walk to the end of the building. Sometimes it was necessary to walk down steps, along a narrow passageway between buildings and under an overhead walkway. I might even have had to cross that walkway to find a flat on the upper section but would first have had to identify the stone steps that led from the ground floor to the first floor. None of this was easy, especially in the dark. The final blow was that only about twenty-five percent of the properties displayed house numbers. One would be forgiven for thinking that the occupants were not keen on visitors' finding their home, whether the caller be the police, social worker or rent collector.

If location was successful, the welcome by the patient and spouse was usually warm and tea was invariably offered. The dog typically joined in the reception party by jumping all over me and licking me to death with an enthusiasm that increased progressively with each command from its owners to cease. Eventually, poor dog would be manhandled into the kitchen where the door would be slammed behind it. The only evidence of its presence thereafter was repetitive barking. I never discovered whether these dogs were simply manic or whether the visit of a hospital consultant was its most exciting experience in months.

The welcome from the inhabitants was indeed warm provided the property was occupied at the time of the visit. Unfortunately, it often wasn't. After two to three minutes' knocking at an unmarked door with no response, a neighbour would hastily appear to act as the Local Information Officer and to tell me that, yes, this was the right house but, no, the ill man requiring my attention was not in but was at work/in the pub/at his mother's/shopping with the missus/gone to fetch the kids (delete as appropriate).

One day, I called to see a middle-aged lady whom the GP had suspected of having a stroke. I knocked at the door and was soon greeted by a smiling, upright lady who was clearly expecting me.

"I've come to see Miss Smithers," I said. "Have I got the right house?"

"Yes, love," she said. "That's me!"

Anybody less looking as if they had had a stroke was hard to imagine but, by now, I had been around long enough to know that medicine loves disguises. We went into the lounge where, after receiving my cup of tea, I enquired about her symptoms. She lived alone. The day before, she had developed sudden paralysis of the right arm and leg and inability to speak for about ten minutes, after which she had recovered completely. She called the doctor who arranged for me to visit the following day. Unbeknown to the GP, on the morning of my visit, the same thing had happened again but for much longer.

"How long did the paralysis last this time?" I asked.

"Well, it started about nine and went on while three."

"Six hours? And what did you do when it happened? Did you call anyone?"

"Oh no, love," she said. "I just stayed on the settee."

"Weren't you worried?"

"Oh no, love. I knew it would get better in the end because it did the day before. Anyway, I couldn't tell no-one, could I, because me voice'd gone."

She burst into laughter at this realisation.

Miss Smithers was another lady with transient ischaemic attacks but this time the blockage was in the main artery to the brain. If we didn't do something soon, she would probably have a major stroke with permanent paralysis. This is probably what the GP had meant from the previous day's experience but his communication had somehow been lost in translation. I explained that she needed to come into hospital urgently.

"Can it wait while tomorrow after I've been to Tesco?" she asked.

"No. I am afraid not."

"Well, I've got bingo tonight. What shall we do about that?"

"Well, I'm not going and I don't think you should either." She laughed.

"All right, love, if you say so. I'll come into your hospital for you today," she said and added with a flourish "And you can do what you will!" She laughed again. "Just you make sure I don't stay in there forever!"

We admitted her to hospital that evening and identified that one of the main arteries in the neck was very narrowed. She had an operation to remove the blockage and recovered well. I saw her in the Outpatient Department six weeks later as a routine follow up.

"Hello, Miss Smithers. How are you?"

"I'm fine, love. But then I always were, weren't I? Your hospital hasn't made me any worse, anyway." She laughed again. Then she added, "Joking apart, I want to thank you and all your staff for everything you have done for me. You have saved my life and the nurses were lovely."

"I don't know about that – I mean the bit about saving lives – but you could have had a nasty stroke."

"I know and thank you. Is that all now? I know you are busy and have more important things to do than pass the time of day with me."

I made a few more checks but then let her go. "Hope I don't see you again," she said and laughed. A lovely lady.

Back at The Ranch (aka the Teaching Hospital), the days were nowhere near as exciting. On the whole, the patients turned up to see me as appointed in the Outpatient Department or on the ward, which, unlike the patients' houses, were both easy to locate because they didn't move from week to week and nobody had removed the signs. Ward rounds, clinics and postgraduate meetings, repeated week after week, can become a little tedious. Without the Doncaster coal fields to amuse us, it was necessary to generate our own fun.

In one respect, becoming a consultant is a champagne-popping moment but, in another, is an anticlimax. The years of competitive goal seeking, the professional treadmill, come to a sudden grinding halt when you realise there is no need for further competition, no more goal to seek. The job henceforward will be secure devotion to healing the sick (or not, as the case may be). Unfortunately, many consultants do not make that transition easily. They fall off the end of the treadmill, stand up, shake themselves down and ask what challenge they can tackle next. Often, if there isn't one in sight, they will manufacture one.

There is usually no reason to pick a fight with the patient, although some patients (or their relatives) are more than ready to take on the doctor. Thus, there are limited outlets for the consultant's challenge culture. Current and historical favourites include management, the heady realms of research and one's colleagues. Manufactured competitive battles may involve one's colleagues because, after all, consultants have spent most of the previous ten years in competition with their peers and some see no good reason to stop. You will find a lot of this sort of people in teaching hospitals.

It is quite some time now since we had simple hospital managers. They evolved progressively through hospital administrators to chief executives. Whether the job has changed significantly over the years is hard to say but the remuneration certainly has. With the money goes the power. Some mentor once told me that there are only two things that motivate people (actually, I think he meant doctors): money and power – in that order. Consultants as a body progressively lost out to management in both money and power stakes.

For people who value money and power, the sight of a manager having a larger salary and increasingly being able to turn the whining consultant at his office door into a servant of the system whose dismissal he can engineer without much difficulty, is galling. The only way to handle this new-found rich, powerful body is to join it, in one form or another. So no longer will you see consultants engaged in clinical care on the one hand and managers in administration on the other but hybrids of the two. The initial consultant coup here was in their perception that they could offer clinical management skills to managers but managers, who are not medically qualified, could not offer clinical skills to consultants.

Recent years have seen a spawning collection of consultant jobs with varying degrees of managerial content, reflected in the acquisition of another title: Medical Director, Assistant Medical Director, Clinical Director for each speciality, Assistant Clinical Director for each speciality, Director of Medical Education. With the new title comes a new grandeur and a step further along the new fabricated professional treadmill. I wouldn't be surprised if we see Junior Assistant Clinical Director for Non-Clinical Matters, Deputy Project Manager of Non-Surgical Input into Impossible Cardiac Surgery or Manager of Monitoring of Management Skills.

Not to be outdone, the "pure" managers are on the fight back for power in the guise of efficiency, an important managerial principle. One manager's proposal, for example, was to limit a particular operating list to one type of operation, thereby avoiding the need for several different sets of specialist surgical equipment and incidentally any decision-making contribution from the consultant. Unfortunately, his approach did not readily cater for emergency or even semi-urgent cases, in other words the planning of operating lists according to clinical priority as used to be done by the surgeons themselves. He did kindly suggest that the non-routine cases could be done by the surgeon on a Sunday morning, if he wanted to.

So now we have examples of operating lists being put together by someone whose previous job was manager of the local TK-Maxx and whose closest exposure to medicine was visiting Boots the Chemist. Of course, I would not dream of suggesting that this system does not work or more specifically that it creates dangers but it is certainly different. One wonders sometimes whether, despite the intrinsic organisational structure of a system, that it functions in spite rather than because of that organisation and its success is more dependent on someone with sense functioning behind the scenes. That is surely true in the case of one doctor I knew whose main managerial responsibility was the organisation of the hospital's outpatient clinics. However, as a pathologist, he had never done a consultant clinic in his life nor indeed dealt with a patient, at least one who was alive.

One day, about two years into the job, I received a call from a Doncaster GP who informed me without delay that he was not calling in a personal capacity but on behalf of the Local Practitioner's Committee, who represented all practices in the area. That sort of introduction, in which the speaker self-transforms from a person to a job, never bodes well. Dr. Savage, a most unfortunate name I felt, was not about to invite me to dinner and bureaucrats rarely contact people to congratulate them on how well things are going.

Dr. Savage, or to be more precise in this context, the Chairman of the Local Practitioner's Committee, brought me up to speed with "a few concerns" of the Committee. That phrase, euphemistic as it usually is, was fortunately accurate on this occasion because their worries revolved not around a rapidly rising death rate from neurological causes focussed on Doncaster but delay in receiving results of tests carried out on patients at Doncaster Royal Infirmary. I explained that the results were posted to my secretary at Sheffield and I regularly wrote to the appropriate GP when I received the results; there were none outstanding as far as I was concerned. Together, we concluded that there was some lag in the system. I promised to look into it.

Boss of the Secretaries was appointed as detective-in-chief on the case. With her usual diplomatic skills, she managed to wind up most of the departments at Doncaster Royal Infirmary by suggesting that they were tardy in sending out the results. Not so, they retorted and indicated that she should return to her ivory tower where she might find the solution to her problem. Even Boss Lady was fearful of taking on the Royal Mail as a potential faulty link in the chain so she had little choice but to do as suggested. A short search of my secretary's desk, carried out without the need for a warrant, revealed a stash of papers detailing the results of tests extending back to the Neolithic era. Poor Girl had apparently not had the time to link up the results with each patient's file, a prerequisite to sending out relevant information to the GP (even consultants cannot remember the clinical details of all their patients so a list of test results is of little value without the file). Poor Girl left soon afterwards and fortunately her successor did not inherit the problem.

Following this experience, I consulted the Deputy Hospital Administrator in Sheffield. I explained the chaos implicit in a system whereby a clinic in Doncaster is effectively administered from Sheffield. I discussed the physical limitations of my registrars in carrying the notes and the excessive number of steps involved between requesting a test on a patient and communicating the result of that test to the GP. "Many a slip twixt cup and lip" I offered and thought of adding my own contribution "and the number of slips is proportionate to the cup-lip distance". However, I realised that proverbs were not her strong point when I saw that her face was as blank as an artist's virgin canvas. I suggested a computer link between the two hospitals and a separate set of notes in Doncaster so results could be accessed directly from the relevant department, appointments could be booked on line and management of the patients' files would not require the services of a haulage operator. Clearly, money would need to be spent, a point that was doubtless not lost on her.

"I don't see how a computer would help you," she said after twenty-nine nanoseconds of reflection.

Sometimes one has to cope without the benefits of managerial input. He who pays the piper calls the tune. A dog is a man's best friend.

One way to maintain dynamism over the years and incidentally to provide a major source of amusement is to superspecialise within the field of neurology, concentrating activities on, say, stroke, epilepsy or multiple sclerosis. I chose movement disorders.

Every man gets a narrower and narrower field of knowledge in which he must be an expert in order to compete with other people. The specialist knows more and more about less and less and finally knows everything about nothing. Konrad Lorenz

One advantage of superspecialisation is that it allows one to avoid seeing conditions that are no longer of interest and maybe never were (such as dizzy spells, which, in my experience, interest nobody, within the field of neurology at least). A development of the tactic is to convince the Department of Neurology and thereafter the funding bodies that we (notice the "we") need a neurologist who specialises in, say, migraine because there is a particular demand in the area/the condition has advanced so much recently that it cannot be dealt with by a generalist/such an appointment would show up the hospital as advanced, forward looking and responsive to the Community/it would generate further resources (delete according to feedback from the person you are trying to persuade). By the way, "resources" in medicine universally means "money".

A second benefit of the approach is that increasing monopolisation of the subspeciality makes you an expert at the local level and nobody else bothers to deal with it any longer. Consultant colleagues become increasingly incapable of questioning your opinion and the longer you work within the specialist area, the less are they likely to do because they increasingly believe that you might actually know something. At postgraduate meetings, what used to be discussions amongst equally informed colleagues now becomes a unilateral display of expertise, justified or not, against a backdrop of fawning ignorance. The effect is enhanced by a measured use of overconfidence. The pinnacle of the development is when all consultants in the department are superspecialised in different areas because each can take their turn as the doyenne scattering pearls of wisdom to the neurological bourgeoisie.

If demand increases so that a second consultant is appointed with the same subspecialist interest, it is essential to demarcate areas within the subspeciality (such as young stroke) that belong to one person and others (such as stroke in the elderly) that belong to the other. This tactic ensures maintenance of the one-man-one-power principle and its immunity from attack by enthusiastic amateurs. I know of one consultant in orthopaedics (the philosophy is not unique to neurology) who was a virtuoso performer of the art. His speciality progressed over the years from general orthopaedics to, within orthopaedics, the shoulder and upper limb, followed by the arm (not shoulder), the wrist and hand, the hand, the fingers and finally the finger joints. I haven't heard of him for some years but can envisage nothing that would have prevented the logical progression to specialisation in the index finger and subsequently index finger (terminal joint). It wouldn't surprise me to learn of his later specialisation, if warranted by forces rallied against his power monopoly, in left (but not right) index finger (terminal joint).

A word of caution: ill-considered deployment of the tactic can leave one vulnerable from a paucity of patients; there is nothing managers love more than an underemployed doctor because it stirs them into action to "Do something!!" about it. So be sure that, in choosing between say left and right index finger (terminal joint), you carry out market research to identify the side with a lot of patients (for you) and the side with no patients (for your colleague). The managers will then recognise his lack of activity and persuade him to take on general cases or engineer his departure to Somewhere Else. Either way, you will retain control of the subspeciality. If you end up with too many patients, you can always see a good proportion privately (superspecialist services attract larger fees which have not so far been affected by the Monopolies Commission).

The final advantage of superspecialisation is that one becomes a member of a worldwide club. The more specialised a subject the fewer the practitioners. Research conferences therefore need to recruit worldwide to generate enough participants and the venue can only reasonably be expected to change from one conference to the next. Thus, interaction with colleagues may entail travelling to far-off lands, such as California, Florida, Venice and Tokyo. By the way, many of these places have Disney theme parks, art galleries or both. And they all have good restaurants.

My movement disorder clinic dealt with tremors, twitches, spasms, unsteadiness and the like in conditions such as Parkinson's disease. One of my colleagues called it the Shakers and Movers Clinic. A patient told me that his workmates called him God because he moved in mysterious ways. The clinic was held every Monday morning. The downside of this arrangement was that it marked a rather nerve-jarring start to the week; much better to spend the first half day of the week deleting emails. The upside was that the physical and psychological debris of a weekend of heavy alcoholic festivity would go unnoticed because the patient's tremor and slurred speech would usually be worse than yours, thereby providing welcome distracting effects.

Nobody, patient or doctor, knows at first whether the presenting symptom will turn out to be a minor irritation or a life sentence.

John Fairburn came to see me one Monday morning. He was a forty-six-year-old joiner who had noticed shaking in his right hand over about the previous three months.

"The funny thing," he said, "is that I don't notice it when I am working. It's only when I get home and rest in the chair that it comes on. My wife says it's the stress of living with her but, if that's right, she doesn't understand why she doesn't have a worse one because she has to live with me." We both laughed. "Seriously though, it is worse when I am stressed – like when I get worked up about something on the telly."

"Most tremors are worse under stress," I explained ,"but that doesn't mean that stress has caused them."

"What this government is doing is enough to make anyone shake."

"Well, that's true," I said. I was tempted to respond in kind but sensed that the depth of shared feeling between us might lead to a lengthy interchange that would eclipse the whole clinic.

"Let's have a look. Just relax."

I moved the hand at the wrist and forearm through the natural excursion of the elbow and wrist joints and sensed a certain stiffness of the muscles, as if moving over a cogwheel. I got him to tap the index finger rapidly and repeatedly against the thumb and saw that the movements were slow and became slower as he continued the tapping. That was enough. Mr. Fairburn had Parkinson's disease.

I now had to explain to him that he had a chemical deficiency in part of his brain, that the condition tended to get worse with time and that there was no cure but treatment was available to put back the missing chemical. However, he didn't need it yet.

In response to direct questions, I answered that, yes, other limbs could be affected; yes, he may have difficulty walking; yes, in time, the treatment may be less effective; yes, there can be side effects of the medication; yes, he may at some point be unable to work. Worse than that, no, I couldn't be precise about timescale because the condition differs a lot between people. But many people go for many years without major problems.

"Well, at least I've got youth on my side" he said. That much was true. But Parkinson's disease tends to be worse in younger people.

Mr. Fairburn would now embark on what has been called "the journey" of years of uncertainty at the significance of some new symptom, whether the new symptom is due to his Parkinson's disease or something else, whether it is a sign of worsening of the condition, whether it can be treated and when and how will his day-to-day life be disrupted. His particular journey brought him, ten years later, to walking with a bent posture and severe shuffle, slurred speech, dribbling of saliva and hallucinations from his medication. He had had to give up work and needed help from his wife to dress, shower and feed. He was on five different drugs for Parkinson's disease.

Parkinson's disease is named after James Parkinson, not because he had it and so it was "his disease" but because he was the first to describe its characteristic features. He described six patients with "shaking palsy" in 1817. Two of them he had met casually in the street and a third he observed only at a distance which all goes to prove that, if you know what you are looking for, it is easy to spot it. This is particularly true of many neurological disorders because the people afflicted often have a characteristic way of moving (or not moving). More than once have I sat in a hotel foyer observing one neurological condition after another pass before my eyes. The experiences tend to provoke feelings that one has missed the turning to the reception area and somehow ended up in a neurology ward or that one is amnesic for the occasion on which a promise had been made to carry out an informal neurology clinic in the hotel.

It is surprising that James Parkinson had time for neurology because he also wrote many articles on other subjects, such as gout, appendicitis and the consequences of being struck by lightning; he wrote a number of books, including one entitled "Hints for the Improvement of Trusses" and others on non-medical subjects, including a compendium of chemistry called "The Chemical Pocket-Book"; he was a staunch activist for political reform, writing under the pseudonym Old Hubert. One article against a political opponent written in 1793 was entitled "An Address to the Honorable Edmund Burke from the Swinish Multitude". On one occasion, James Parkinson was summoned to give evidence concerning a plot to assassinate the King, although he was not himself on trial, which is just as well because a guilty verdict would have brought a rapid end to his days on earth and no book on Parkinson's disease.

This eclectic catalogue of interests beats in depth and variety the extracurricular interests of most modern neurologists. James Parkinson also differed in another important respect from many of today's specialists: he was modest. His monograph introduces his observations with the statement that "some conciliatory explanation should be offered for the present publication: in which, it is acknowledged, that mere conjecture takes the place of experiment." He felt that "to delay...publication did not appear warrantable" because "the disease had escaped particular notice" but hoped that "the offering of the following pages to the attention of the medical public will not be severely censured." To be fair to modern neurologists, maybe everyone spoke and wrote like that. Or not.

It would appear that James Parkinson didn't have time for neurological niceties and homed in on key facts. He was clearly not a follower of the philosophy that the more academic irrelevances are incorporated into an analysis of a clinical problem, the more impressive is the display of neurological expertise (this is a technique known, in the medical profession, as hoodwinking).

Nobody is really sure to what extent Parkinson's disease existed before James Parkinson (well, clearly not at all by that name, anyway) and, if not, what brought it into existence, barring the will of God and malign extraterrestrial influences. Some people blame James Stephenson who invented the railway – well, perhaps not literally, but at least the industrial revolution and its associated environmental pollution and life before the Clean Air Act 1956. By this notion, the Victorians designed not only heavy industry but also some cute human diseases based upon one or other form of poisoning.

Sceptics beware! In the nineteenth century, hat makers used to use a mercury solution in a process of curing animal pelts. As a result of poor ventilation in the workshop, the hatters breathed in the toxic fumes and developed mercury poisoning. The effects on the nervous system included tremors (hatter's shakes), poor coordination, numbness and weakness in the hands and feet, slurred speech, visual difficulty, anxiety and hallucinations. Mercury was responsible for being "as mad as a hatter".

People, on the whole, are slow learners: despite knowledge of the nineteenth-century disease, many people in Japan suffered similar problems from eating shellfish and other fish contaminated with methylmercury from the industrial effluent of the Chisso Corporation Chemical Factory in the late twentieth century. It is rumoured that, despite continuing deaths and disability, neither the Government nor the Company did much to prevent the pollution. The reason for any delay in acting is not clear but I imagine has little to do with economic, capitalist or profit-making considerations.

At the time of writing, it is regarded amongst the cogniscenti as politically incorrect to talk about Parkinson's disease because "disease" has connotations of contamination and contagion. Terms such as Parkinson's disorder or even just Parkinson's are preferred to avoid the stigma. I have always thought the latter proposal was unfortunate for at least two reasons: first, it is a cliff-hanger because we never learn to what the genitive case of Parkinson refers; and, secondly, the abbreviation seems somehow to increase Parkinson's responsibility for the disease in crediting him with an ownership interest in everyone afflicted with the condition when his only involvement was its recognition and description.

We have seen similar naming problems in other conditions: thus Mongolism became Downs syndrome; cretinism became infantile hypothyroidism; disabled became disadvantaged. All these changes of name are valiant efforts to avoid the social stigma associated with the particular condition. Sadly, people do not change and the stigma soon catches up with the relabelling once the stigmatiser realises that the name, but not the nature of the affliction, has changed. The Oxford English Dictionary tells us that "disease" comes from the old French "desaise" meaning "lack of ease" or "inconvenience" whereas "disorder" in medicine is "an illness that disrupts normal physical or mental function". You would think that "disease" was less pejorative based on these definitions, but there we are.

What's in a name? That which we call a rose by any other name would smell as sweet.   William Shakespeare "Romeo and Juliet"

Talking of names, another common cause of tremor is known as benign essential tremor, "essential" because it is regarded as an inherent system fault and "benign" because it does not produce a serious disability as can Parkinson's disease. It usually causes shaking of the hands when trying to do something such as holding a cup and saucer. It is probably the biggest single cause of the Grandma-is-Coming Syndrome, the audible rattle of the cup on the saucer that heralds her arrival from the kitchen with the afternoon tea. (Do not google this syndrome. I made it up. However, benign essential tremor really is real. Come to think of it, Grandma-is-Coming Syndrome is quite a good name for a syndrome – I might work on it.) The tremor is improved dramatically but temporarily by alcohol, a fact which probably explains why Bill Werbeniuk was often deemed to be intoxicated when playing his best snooker.

Jay Fleet, aged thirty-four, came to see me with shaking of the hands. She had benign essential tremor. I tried treatment with beta-blocking drugs, which often works, but it was only partially effective in her case. She was a professional golfer and had to give up her career. It appears that golf is more affected by alcohol intoxication than is snooker.

For a sedentary man or woman, benign essential tremor may cause little inconvenience apart from rattling of the newspaper but, for a professional sportsperson or musician, it can be a blast out of the career water.

Ruth Henson, aged fifty-six, also had shaking of the hands due to benign essential tremor. She had never drunk alcohol in her life but, six months earlier, someone had told her that a small glass of sherry taken before a social outing, when the tremor embarrassed her most, would probably help. Within six months, she was drinking a bottle of vodka per day.

Not for these two ladies was the tremor "benign".

An alternative to superspecialisation as a method of maintaining control of one's area of work is the invention of a new speciality with, of course, its own dedicated clinic. One of the best examples I have come across is a clinic specialising in the investigation and treatment of the neurologically obscure. The founder of this service played a masterstroke by devoting himself to management of what are almost by definition the more difficult cases in neurology whilst at the same time focussing on what is probably undiagnosable and untreatable. The altruism inherent in dealing, by choice, with difficult work gains brownie points from one's colleagues and other consultants are unlikely to be critical of failure to solve a problem that has eluded everyone else. Indeed, wise policy is not to solve most of these clinical obscurities, even if it were possible to do so, for fear of casting a shadow of failure over the consultant or consultants who previously assessed the case.

I was tempted to this notion after a general neurology outpatient clinic where I saw a man with back pain. Three weeks previously, he had come to see me, complaining of the sudden onset of pain to the right side of his lumbar spine two weeks before. The pain had come on when he was lifting his wife's wheelchair into the van and had shot down his right leg. It had persisted despite bed rest advised by the GP. His wife had had to stop using her wheelchair and walk instead because nobody was available to get it out of the van. Quite why she needed the wheelchair in the first place is another question and one that was never quite answered but, over the two-week period, she had been on her feet looking after her husband and was worn out.

I suspected he had had an attack of sciatica from a slipped disc in his back and sent him for an MRI scan which indeed confirmed a small disc prolapse at the appropriate level. He returned to the clinic with his wife, who, to my amazement, was now back in her wheelchair and he seemed to be pushing it without difficulty.

"All the pain has gone," he said excitedly. "It went all of a sudden yesterday morning."

I was about to explain that sciatica can get better on its own, often fairly quickly, but his wife had had other ideas.

"I am fairly sure now", she said, "that it was trapped wind. When the wind was released, the pain went."

I agreed that excess wind in the bowel can cause a colicky abdominal pain but it could hardly produce pain on one side of the back going down the leg to the ankle. I did not enquire in too much detail the circumstances of the release of wind sufficient to ease pain that had rendered him immobile for two weeks.

She went on: "I don't know if you know, doctor, but trapped wind can show itself in very many guises."

At that moment, the idea crystallised: all my cases of headache, visual disturbance, dizzy spells, blackouts, back pain, numbness and more could all be transferred to my newly founded Trapped Wind Clinic, all to be instantly cured by the generation of one big fart.

An alternative source of amusement for a hospital consultant is the system of merit awards which are granted on a discretionary basis for exceptional clinical services. Before the launch of the National Health Service in 1948, the Spens Committee reported on the Remuneration of Consultants and Specialists. One of its recommendations was that there should be additions to the basic specialist salary to provide incentive and to reward outstanding work. A cynic might suggest that an ulterior motive was to ensure active involvement of all specialists in the new national service and no-one could afford to let a simple matter of income prevent recruitment of the filthy rich but I know of no evidence for (or, for that matter, against) that proposition. Three levels of award were suggested.

In the British Medical Journal of June 12 1948, the leader writer commented on the awards as follows: "The Committee then goes on to the most controversial of its recommendations in its suggestion that these awards shall be made by a national committee, the professional members of which are to be nominated by the Royal Colleges and the Scottish Royal Corporations, having among its members a representative of the Universities and of the Medical Research Council. Consultants and specialists should scrutinize this recommendation with care. ...... The procedure contemplated will be open to abuse, even though such abuse might not be evident to the committee in session. We believe it is inadvisable that a central committee composed largely of specialists should be given this financial control over all specialists working in the National Health Service. Will the committee at its first meeting debar its own members from these awards?"

"It is to be hoped that the consultants and specialists generally will voice their opinions on this procedure, which is the one outstandingly unsatisfactory proposal in a report which is likely to commend itself to those who will work as consultants and specialists in the new Service." As far as I know, nobody objected - at least, nobody with any influence because the system went ahead.

Nine years later, on 25 March 1957, a debate took place in the House of Commons. Mr. John Peyton, MP for Yeovil, asked the Minister of Health on what basis merit awards were made to consultants; by whom such awards were recommended; and to what extent regional hospital boards who had to meet the cost were consulted. He was told that thirty-four percent of consultants received awards valued from five hundred pounds to two thousand five hundred pounds per year on the recommendations of an advisory committee;

regional hospital boards were not consulted. Mr. Peyton asked for wider knowledge of how the committee made its awards but was told that "the whole idea of the awards is that they are on a professional basis". In other words, they are decided by consultants in secret.

Mrs. Bessie Braddock pointed out that the details of those who obtained awards used to be submitted to the management committees of hospitals and that that had ceased to be done. She was told that the change was made "in the interests of patients and not necessarily of the consultants concerned". In other words, it makes no difference to the people who pay for the awards to be told who is receiving them but it would mean a patient would suffer by knowing that their consultant was being paid more than somebody else's. If you believe that, you will believe anything.

The Minister of Health promised to look again at the issue but felt that the disadvantages of doing what Bessie proposed would outweigh the advantages. Quite why is not stated.

The following year, on 8 December 1958, a further debate took place. Mr. Ellis Smith, MP for Stoke-on-Trent South, wanted to know how much money was paid to consultants under the merit award scheme but was told by the Minister of Health that the information was not available. The Minister of Health felt regret about it but not half as much, it appears, as did Mr. Smith who thought that operation of a merit scheme in secret was what politicians call A Decidedly Bad Idea. Dr. Edith Summerskill, MP for Warrington, pointed out that this might be the only case where public money was spent without knowing how much or why but was told that the scheme had continued to date because it had given broad satisfaction, "at any rate to the profession concerned" and no-one had found a satisfactory alternative method. So that's all right, then.

An editorial in The Independent on 16 January 1998 pointed out a recent study published in the British Medical Journal which found that fourteen percent of consultants were non-white but only five percent of them held a distinction award and referred to previous studies which showed that men were more likely to receive an award than women; the specialties of cardiology and surgery were favoured over psychiatry and geriatrics; and academics in teaching hospitals received more awards than ordinary working doctors in district hospitals.

The awards were said to be given "solely on grounds of merit but ... they are not intended - nor should they be seen - as a measure of the quality of treatment afforded to individual patients". Being a good doctor does not earn Brownie points, unfortunately, at least not when traded in for money.

The Guardian, on 7 November 2002, reported a study from the Medical Practitioners' Union and stated: "White consultants in England and Wales were three times more likely than those from ethnic minorities to get distinction awards, which can add up to £62,815 a year to their salaries."

"In obstetrics and gynaecology, dermatology and general surgery, the chances of a white consultant getting an award last year were ten times greater than those of an ethnic minority colleague."

"In trauma and orthopaedics, the white consultant surgeon was thirty times more likely to be given an award by one of the regional committees who govern the allocations."

"Among 1,000 white consultants in trauma and orthopaedics, there were 106 with distinction awards, but, among 254 from ethic minorities, there was only one with an award."

"The study also showed male consultants were twice as likely to be given an award as female consultants."

On 25 March 1999, the Health Service Journal stated that four unnamed consultants would lose merit awards, each worth £24,640 annually because they had "not continued to fulfil the criteria" under a new five-yearly review system. The criteria do not seem to be obvious.

Until then, merit awards, once given, were never removed so the recipient retained the increased salary until retirement. Since the consultant's pension was salary-dependent, he or she would also benefit from an enhanced pension. However, James Wisheart, who was struck off by the

General Medical Council the previous year after an inquiry into baby deaths at Bristol Royal Infirmary, continued to receive the benefits of his A award (the second highest). James Wisheart was found guilty of serious professional misconduct over the deaths of twenty-nine babies following heart surgery.

All in all, a very satisfactory system, it seemed. Or not.

Things have improved in recent years but, in the 1980s and 1990s, the system was about as negotiable, transparent and above board as a Yorkshire coalface in the dark. One Wednesday afternoon, having been allocated an award the previous year, I was allowed to attend the meeting that would decide who was to receive awards in the current year. As I entered the lecture theatre where the meeting was held, my first focus of attention was the rows of other consultants present, all of whom must have had an award to be allowed into the meeting and whose identity had until then been about as well known as the workings of GCHQ.

The meeting was officially chaired by a manager. However, seated on the front row, with self-assumed authority, was one of the professors of medicine who maintained constant eye contact with the chairman throughout the proceedings. He effectively directed the whole programme, seemingly through a combination of choice facial expression, perfectly timed vocal interjection and probably an element of hypnosis as well. It certainly seemed as if the only notes taken by the chairman were in response to something communicated directly or indirectly by this man.

"We have had proposals for C awards for Dr. Forrest from Cardiology and Dr. Jenkins from Radiology. We only have one award available at this stage so we will have to choose between the two" explained the chairman. No response from Golden Eagle on the front row.

The chairman went on to summarise the CVs of the two candidates, both of whom sounded as if they should be given fifty merit awards, not one. I thought of suggesting that they be referred for canonisation as the patron saints of hearts and X-rays but decided the remark might be perceived as flippant. I cannot remember the details exactly now but Dr. Jenkins had done something like designing a form of X-ray that could be processed in fresh water streams in Somalia and Dr. Forrest had developed a cardiac intervention unit, housed in a new hospital extension. All funding for the venture had been raised by the cardiologist who, for all I know, built the extension with his own bare hands as well. Anyway, it was all pretty impressive stuff.

Many of the assembled company spoke out with carefully considered appraisal of the relative merits of the two consultants. The X-ray innovation had the merit of international recognition but was not really serving the

National Health Service whereas the cardiac unit was a clinical facility that had not yet reached its full potential. There was almost universal agreement, however, that Dr. Forrest, the cardiologist, had made the major contribution and deserved the award.

Golden Eagle stirred. "I don't really know him," he said, "but I have worked closely with Dr. Jenkins for some years and he is a very good radiologist."

The chairman sought to highlight the parts of the CVs that had led most of the audience to favour the cardiologist's contribution to that of the radiologist.

"I understand the unit is a state-of-the-art facility with only three others in Europe able to offer equivalent resources to cardiac patients," he said.

"Hand on heart," said Eagle, "I would prefer Dr. Jenkins."

"Shouldn't it be hand on X-ray?" said the chairman and burst into uncontrollable giggling. Unfortunately, few others, and certainly not Golden Eagle, saw the funny side. His laughter ceased abruptly on sensing the penetrating stare and telepathic waves emanating from the front row.

By now, most of the audience had lapsed into a quiescent apathy, realising that their corporate thoughts had gained their representation in the chairman's voice. Essentially, it was now all down to him and Eagle.

"I have got to know Dr. Jenkins very well," said Eagle, "and have little doubt that he deserves an award. I find Dr. Forrest a little complacent. He has certainly never discussed his project with me, which I find surprising." (Quite why it was surprising, since he was in a different department, escaped me.)

Eagle went on to explain, inter alia, that Dr. Jenkins had often discussed his radiology plans with him over a drink by the pool or when shooting a few holes at Sickleholme Golf Club.

Towards the end of his monologue, I noticed that a few members of the audience had fallen asleep and most of the rest appeared to be in a state of suspended animation, all critical faculties suspended.

"Dr. Forrest is altogether too much of an unknown quantity," he said with a tone of finality. The chairman closed the meeting. The audience woke up. The contingent dispersed back into anonymity. Dr. Jenkins got his award.

The executioner's face is always well hidden. Bob Dylan "A Hard Rain's Gonna Fall"

Most hospital doctors were on call at nights and weekends to deal with emergencies and acute admissions but the nature of the task differed with the seniority of the post. The junior grades, who could be said to work on the front line, were likely to be actively working in the hospital during an on-call period and would get little sleep. If they did, it was likely to be for a couple of hours in a hospital on-call room, which could scarcely be called home from home. For a consultant, at least in neurology, the on-call was usually taken at home, which in one respect was preferable. However the arrangement prompted two sword analogies: first, the double-edged one because the comfort of being at home was offset by having to get up, dress and drive into the hospital where necessary – much easier to be on the premises. It is also easier to avoid alcohol in hospital than at home. The second sword was the Damocles one, which hung over the head with the potential to fall unpredictably and with uncertain consequences – mere telephone advice or the dreaded midnight trip to hospital?

I did work as a registrar for one consultant who managed to control the system to fit his own requirements. On one occasion, for example, I telephoned to give the details of a new admission but was intercepted by his wife who advised me to call back in about twenty minutes because my mentor was watching University Challenge. That response would not have gone down well in my days as a consultant but, to be fair, there were fewer treatable neurological disorders in his day so he no doubt felt, probably correctly in his case, that little would be gained by interrupting his TV schedule.

The Damocles effect is considerably enhanced at Christmas when the stakes are much higher. Sacrifice of locally reared turkey and premier cru claret to a hospital intrusion is profoundly more emotionally damaging than loss of a Tesco burger, even one from its Finest range. Consultants routinely saw all the acute cases within twenty-four hours of admission, depending upon the urgency, so a certain amount of social planning was essential at the best of times. At Christmas, this requirement, and the associated disruption to the family party, was best offset by a planned trip into the ward on Christmas morning to deliver the ward present, eat mince pies, kiss the nurses and, if time permitted, to see the patients as well before returning home for lunch. An anaesthetic dose of sherry provided by the ward sister ("Go on, its Christmas!") facilitated the whole process.

But sometimes the most careful planning can be sidestepped by a neurological condition determined to cause maximum inconvenience. One Christmas Eve, we were winding down the ward in preparation for Christmas, employing various traditional seasonal tactics, such as lowering the threshold for hospital discharge, when, at 5 p.m. on the nail, I received a call from a district general hospital.

"Dr. Sagar, we have a very ill patient here. We think he has tetanus. We would like to transfer him to you as an emergency."

A few essential questions probed the possibility that the call represented an example of shuffling off of responsibility by the referring doctors in preparation for

Christmas but their answers increasingly showed that I was unlikely to find a plausible excuse not to accept the patient. First, the patient had only been admitted that morning. Secondly, there was little evidence that they had exaggerated his symptoms for effect and, thirdly, he had worsened suddenly that afternoon. Try as I might, I could not escape the conclusion that the referral was right on two accounts: the man was very ill and he had tetanus. Their third point, that he should be transferred to our care, seemed impossible to refute despite many years of experience in the exercise.

Tetanus is caused by infection of a wound with Clostridium tetani, a bacterium which secretes toxin into the blood stream. This toxin causes intense muscle spasm throughout the body, often beginning in the jaw ("lockjaw"). At its peak, the spasms are so great that huge strain is placed upon other organs, including the heart and kidneys. Dealing with these problems takes hours of continuous treatment, monitoring and interception. There would be no sleep that Christmas Eve, I knew. I finally got home at 11 a.m. on Christmas morning, having had to forgo the ward festivities. I didn't even feel like kissing the nurses. I was back in hospital late on Christmas Day and for most of Boxing Day. Tetanus is not much fun, even for the patient.

The ability to make a sensible assessment at the end of the telephone obviously depends on the quality of the information conveyed. Most of the time, junior staff are remarkably adept at conveying the essence of the problem, bearing in mind that they have had no training in public speaking and probably less than ten years earlier were rendered virtually mute by a state of chronic adolescent stupor. It is amazing what happens when a few brain cells connect.

John McIntyre was different. He could communicate well and was usually right in his assessments but he chose to withhold key pieces of information in the manner of a television detective drama, a tactic used to enhance suspense in the viewer. When asked a specific question, he would respond either in joyous confirmation of my insight or by considered provision of another relevant fragment of evidence.

"We have a forty-two-year-old man admitted with paralysis of his right side." Silence.

"Did it come on suddenly?"

"No! Over about two hours." Further silence.

"Does he have a high temperature?"

"YES, HE DOES!!"

"What do *you* think is the diagnosis?" I asked.

"I think he has encephalitis."

"I agree."

On another occasion: "We have a thirty-eight-year-old woman admitted with paralysis of the left limbs," he began and added, almost as an afterthought, "Came on suddenly", obviously with the intention of directing me towards the diagnosis of stroke, the commonest cause of acute paralysis of one side of the body.

"Is there any significant past history?" I asked.

"She has rheumatoid arthritis," he said. His voice lowered in pitch by about an octave and halved in tempo as he spoke the words "rheumatoid arthritis". He waited for my response.

"Do we have any blood results?"

"Her ESR is up at seventy-five."

"That could be because her arthritis is active. Does it seem so clinically?" I asked.

"N o-o-o," he said ponderously but expectantly.

"Or she may have a vasculitis," (inflammation of the blood vessels, leading to thrombosis and stroke and associated with some other conditions, such as rheumatoid arthritis).

"YES!" he said explosively.

Brian Butterworth was also excited about neurology and enigmatic in his presentations.

"We have had a twenty-five-year-old girl admitted with progressive weakness and numbness of both legs over a period of two weeks."

He explained that the reflexes in both legs were exaggerated and we agreed that she probably had a lesion of the spinal cord. At her age and with the speed of progression, the diagnosis was probably transverse myelitis due to inflammation within the spinal cord.

"Are there any signs outside the spinal cord?" I asked.

"She has bilateral optic pallor." The last three words, which indicate damage to the nerves controlling vision, were uttered at a pitch and tempo remarkably similar to those adopted by Dr. McIntyre on such occasions.

He was excited by his finding because the combination of optic nerve damage and myelitis usually indicates a diagnosis of multiple sclerosis, as opposed to other causes of spinal cord damage. When I saw the notes, I found that he had even written the words "bilateral optic pallor" in block capitals, underlined and followed by three exclamation marks. The diagnosis "multiple sclerosis" had a similar font style.

Brian Butterworth resembled John McIntyre in his confidence and presentation style but differed in one important respect: Brian was almost always wrong. There was no optic pallor and she did not have multiple sclerosis. I wished I could have curbed his enthusiasm but it was to no avail: this pattern of behaviour was to continue for many months until he finally left. I do not know what happened to him – he went off to do a job in psychiatry and hasn't been heard of since.

He's sure got a lotta gall to be so useless an' all. Bob Dylan "Visions of Johanna"

Tuesday and Friday mornings were devoted to ward rounds in which the consultant tours the patients under his care with a variably sized retinue of junior doctors, nurses and students, depending upon who feels like turning up. By now, things had changed a bit since I was a junior doctor. As a surgical houseman, I witnessed the preparations for the ward round, which included all the patients obligatorily changing into their nightwear, even if the ward round was in the early afternoon, and getting into bed. Until ordered otherwise, they were to adopt a semi-sitting, semi-lying posture so that they could communicate readily with the consultant when their turn came and yet transfer readily into a fully supine position should examination be required. I suspect most of them were terrified to move for fear of incurring the sister's wrath - or, to be more precise, her opinion, often forcibly delivered, on the merits or otherwise of doing anything even modestly different from that recommended by her.

The ward was spotless; all used and unnecessary utensils were moved into the sluice; the curtains were opened to exactly three-quarters of the span of the window and carefully adjusted; all nonessential personnel were ejected from the ward and transferred to tasks that kept them quiet and out of the public view (which, in this case, equated to the consultant's view). The ward was of so-called Nightingale type in which all the beds were arranged in sequence down two sides of a large open room so all thirty patients, bedded and in identical, motionless postures, were at once visible from the door. As a consequence of the fastidious preparations, the consultant, on his grand entry to the ward, was confronted by a scene reminiscent of a five-star sanitised sanitorium in which the only way he could possibly distinguish motionless but live patients from dead ones was from information provided by the slightly fawning ward sister.

The consultant's word was final. Patients were allowed (but not encouraged) to ask questions. However, whilst the presumably more important ones, such as, "When will my operation be?" may well have been answered in detail by the consultant, with precise provision of the date and time of surgery, the apparently lesser ones, such as, "Will this cure my problem?" received a more limited response, usually, "Yes", followed by a hasty promise from the ward sister that she would explain everything later. I don't remember anyone asking how long they had to live. Too trivial.

Despite this twice-weekly medical equivalent of a son-et-lumiere spectacle, it was the sister who really owned the ward. The obsessive-compulsive aspects of her ward management (and that of most other ward sisters I met then) underpinned clean, healthy nursing practice. And she knew all her patients in detail. And made sure the other nurses did too. And cared.

Over the decades, the autonomy of the ward sister has been supplanted by one or more forms of nursing management structure, which essentially translates into patient management by committee. This, of course, is often no management at all. One early feature of the process was introduction of the Number Sevens. These nurse managers were so-called because each nursing grade was numbered; sisters were number six and they were one cut above. It is always difficult to judge someone else's profession but, as far as I could see, the Number Sevens spent most of the time walking from ward to ward with a clipboard cradled in the left arm. It was never very clear what resulted from this activity. The doubtless benefit never seemed to emerge from the shadows for long enough to enlighten my ignorance. Anyway, I used to understand ward sisters.

On the whole, nurses did turn up for ward rounds but with just enough uncertainty to raise the anxiety levels. Sadly, they explained, it was impossible to guarantee the sister's attendance on every ward round because of other commitments. Apparently, the ward round and other events could clash sometimes but not always, even though the timings of the two did not vary from week to week. Nurses of lower grade had to be delegated but, since they had almost always just got back after "days off", they were limited in their knowledge of the patients to that written on the crib sheet carried prominently in two hands in front of them.

I believe the information on the sheets was extracted from the nursing notes, which, like all patient records, was required to be accurate, comprehensive and up-to-date. The principle was admirable but the all-inclusive nature of the documentation could lead to provision of much gratuitous comment. Often have I read that Mr. X was made comfortable and attention was given to all his immediate needs but never that Mr. Y was made uncomfortable and his needs were ignored. If the modern press is to be believed, the latter can sometimes now happen but still, for some reason, is never recorded. I am sure ward sisters, especially those longer in the tooth, tolerated the new arrangements with chagrin. The more junior nurses had never known anything else, better or worse, and, pleased to be in The Caring Profession, thought all was hunky-dory.

The usual pattern on ward rounds was to start off in the ward office where the patients could be discussed in their absence, thereby sparing them the emotional trauma of overhearing details of which particular part of their nervous system was rotting away and why. In an attempt to make the students wanted, it was customary to combine the business of the ward round with teaching, usually by intermittently breaking off the conversation with the nurse and junior doctors to interrogate the young medical hopefuls on aspects of neurology relevant to the particular case. When the questions prompted an incorrect answer, the consultant was able to demonstrate his encyclopaedic knowledge by responding with fascinating neurological facts about any condition that was presented before him. When a correct answer was given, the usual technique was to acknowledge its accuracy and then to provide a short monologue which essentially paraphrased the information provided by the student. The main advantage of this strategy was that the consultant always had the last word, whether or not the student was knowledgeable. When students were being taught, the nurses looked bored and, when the patients were discussed, the students looked bored. Junior doctors displayed a constant air that combined appearances of boredom, stress and fatigue.

Most students learn by passive assimilation, their brains adapting to the new clinical world as a young child does to the real world. The inflexible student, however, is a rare but characteristic variant of the species who is keen, knowledgeable, inquiring, faintly aggressive and never bored. This creature asks a lot of questions and finds it difficult to accept that clinical medicine does not always fit the rules. New facts have to fit in with old facts.

"If this patient has a problem in the neck causing entrapment of the seventh cervical nerve root, why do they not have weakness of the triceps muscle which is supplied by that nerve?" he asks.

"They do have weakness of the other muscles supplied by the seventh root and loss of sensation that corresponds with the damage."

"But why not weakness of the triceps?"

"Because the muscle has been spared."

"How?"

"Probably because the parts of the nerve - the nerve fibres - that supply that muscle have not been damaged in the way that the others have."

"But if the whole nerve has been compressed, surely all the fibres would be affected."

"Maybe the fibres to the triceps muscle are more resistant."

"But how?"

These conversations usually ended by my saying something along the lines of "I don't know exactly but, believe me, it happens", the inquisitorial student looking perplexed and disbelieving and the other students rolling their eyes and looking at their watch.

Following this preparatory entertainment, those of us who had not managed to escape between leaving the office and entering the ward, which seemed invariably to include me, went to visit the patients to question, to examine, to explain and even sometimes to diagnose and treat. And so concludes another medical jamboree.

The second round of the week was better than the first because its ending was timed to merge seamlessly with the start of the drive home to the hi-fi and the first gin and tonic of the weekend.

Yes, to dance beneath the diamond sky with one hand waving free, silhouetted by the sea, circled by the circus sands, with all memory and fate driven deep beneath the waves, let me forget about today until tomorrow. Bob Dylan "Mr. Tambourine Man"

Chapter 9: Pesticides, nutrients and other health-giving chemicals

I will lift mine eyes unto the pills. Almost everyone takes them, from the humble aspirin to the multi-coloured, king-sized three deckers, which put you to sleep, wake you up, stimulate and soothe you all in one. It is an age of pills.
Malcolm Muggeridge

Poisons are only poisons if you are sensitive to poisons.

On one of the darker days of December, when the full force of seasonal affective disorder was pushing my mood level to a new low for the year, I had seen a series of difficult patients during the morning and was coming to the conclusion that the outpatient clinic was the worst thing since sliced bread. Shortly afterwards, I found myself face to face with a portly lady, fifty-five years of age, dressed in tight leggings with red and green horizontal stripes, bedecked with daffodil yellow shoes and covered with a tight-fitting gold satin dress that did little to conceal her ample bosom and the abdominal protuberance beneath. Her hair was thick, shoulder length and peroxide blonde and her pouting lips were an unsubtle shade of pink. The necklace resembled a Lord Mayor's chain in purple. The whole colour scheme was enough to provoke a migraine attack in anyone susceptible.

Her curt response of "Hello" to my introductory "Good morning, I am Doctor Sagar, pleased to meet you, do come in and take a seat", accompanied by a visual scan of the room that made her look as if she were searching for explosives or bugging devices, and a total lack of smile, led me, possibly prejudicially, to the conclusion that the consultation might not prove straightforward and any shift in my mood level was unlikely to be upward.

Mrs. Schofield told me that her general practitioner did not understand her problem because, despite numerous attempts at treatment, her condition had persisted. The letter of referral from him had helped me somewhat, at least in understanding that she had recurrent pins and needles on one side of the face. Indeed, without that, I would have lost ten minutes of the consultation without learning anything from the afflicted lady, except that her doctor was unlikely to be medically qualified, or words to that effect.

At a suitable pause in her pronouncement of judgement, which occurred only because she had one thing in common with the rest of the human race, which was the need to breathe, I interjected.

"I see that you have seen a number of consultants previously and they all agree that the pins and needles are not due to anything serious. None of the tests has shown up anything. That is not to say that you do not have these sensations but sometimes we cannot identify the exact cause, short of taking out part of the nerve and putting it under the microscope, which I think would be a bit drastic in your case. I will obviously have another look but, if I cannot find anything either, it is a matter of taking medication that dampens down the feelings without getting at the root cause."

She stiffened in her seat and said, "If I have a fault with my car, I take it back to the dealer and expect it to be fixed. What's the difference?"

I was tempted to say that, unlike the manufacturer of her car, her creator had not provided a design manual but, as usual on such occasions, felt it might be counterproductive. In fact, a little more discussion revealed that she knew the problem was unlikely to be cured permanently and she would have to keep on taking tablets.

"None of them works," she pronounced.

"Do any of the medications help at all?" I asked.

"No, none of them takes away the feelings completely."

"I understand", I said, "but do any help in any way at all?"

"Not completely."

This question-and-answer couplet continued in one form or another for a few more cycles before I was able to establish that some drugs had given partial benefit.

"The white ones helped a bit," she told me.

"Which white ones?" I asked. "Do you know the name of the medication?"

"You know", she said, "the little white tablets."

"There are many drugs that come as little white tablets. Do you know which one it was?"

"As I told you", she answered tersely, "they were little white tablets. If you don't know what they are, how do you expect me to?"

"I will find out from your doctor. Did any others help? What else has been tried?"

"The blue ones were not much use although they were better than the red ones. Mind you, I don't know why he prescribed red ones in the first place. Red tablets never suit me. I'm much better off with white tablets. I told him that when he gave me red antibiotics for a water infection and he ended up having to give me another prescription for white ones. Still, he insisted that we should try red tablets for this face thing. And, of course, they didn't work."

She took a breath which gave me a chance.

"Sometimes the same medicine can come in different coloured tablets," I explained. "It depends to some extent on the company that makes them. One will produce red tablets but another may put the same drug in white tablets. Occasionally the two preparations are not identical but it is not the colour itself that is important."

"Exactly! I told you they were different which is why I always ask for white tablets," she announced. After a barely discernible pause, she continued, "Anyway, when he did eventually get me on white tablets, I started on one a day but, when I got a repeat prescription, I found I had been given two a day. Look, I've kept the packets to prove it. When I can calm myself enough to face that surgery without blowing my top, I am going to show him so that he might at least learn from his mistakes and avoid doing the same to someone else. If I were not so lucky as to know about these things, I could have ended up taking twice the amount that I should have."

"It's all right, Mrs. Schofield", I explained after inspecting the packets. "The ones you were prescribed the second time were half the strength of your first prescription so, by taking two a day, you were taking the same daily dose as the first ones that you took just once per day. I don't know why you were given different strengths but it does not make any difference. You were on the same dose each day with the second prescription as you were with the first."

"How can two tablets a day be the same as one?" she sneered.

Despite another fifteen minutes' conversation, we achieved little common ground. I hope I did my best but I know that, in her mind, I failed.

I'd forever talk to you but soon my words would turn into a meaningless ring for, deep in my heart, I know there's no help I can bring. Bob Dylan "To Ramona"

For a physician, one of the mainstays of treatment is the use of drugs. These days, there is a vast array of drugs available to cure or ameliorate most medical conditions. But it was not always so. Before the 1940s, when penicillin was developed, there were few antibiotics, which were not very powerful, so many people died of infection.

Incidentally, Alexander Fleming is usually credited with the discovery of penicillin. This is technically true but his paper in the British Journal of Experimental Pathology in 1929 was entitled "On the Antibacterial Action of Cultures of a Penicillium with Special Reference to their Use in the Isolation of B. Influenzae" (*B. Influenzae i*s a bacterium). Towards the end of the article, Fleming acknowledges that penicillin had "a possible use in the treatment of bacterial infections" by "application to or injection into areas infected with penicillin-sensitive microbes" but the chemical was "certainly useful to the bacteriologist" for the isolation of certain bacteria in the laboratory.

If he appreciated the real potential value of penicillin in the treatment of human infection, it was arguably not obvious from that paper. It was up to Lord Florey, in Oxford, to carry out trials of the drug in human infection, although, according to him, he was driven by the science and not by human suffering. Florey received the Nobel Prize with Fleming in 1945. One person, who was involved in testing out the drug, told me as a student that the ward was metaphorically split in two with patients on one side treated with penicillin and those on the other receiving only existing treatments. It became so obvious that the penicillin-treated people were doing better that the trial was abandoned, presumably before the ward became only half full.

Nowadays, there are extensive regulatory procedures in place before a drug can be brought to market. Trials in animals are followed by extensive trials in humans which can take many years to complete. All this activity costs a lot of money so the pharmaceutical company responsible for the drug development has to be fairly confident of the outcome of an experimental drug. Even so, a large number of drug projects are begun and abandoned because they do not live up to expectations. Needless to say, the company wants its money back. And people wonder why modern drugs are so expensive.

The nature of treatment has also changed. People were used to taking a course of tablets to treat a condition, usually an infection. The expectation was that this would cure the problem permanently once the course of treatment had finished. However, many modern treatments merely keep the problem at bay. Treatments for diabetes, epilepsy and high blood pressure, for example, only work as long as the medication is taken. If it is stopped, the seizures, high blood glucose or high blood pressure recur. This concept is now commonplace to most people who work in medicine although it did not stop a friend of mine being telephoned in the night by a nurse with the question "Mr. Jones' blood pressure is now normal. Can I therefore stop his treatment?" I don't expect he would have been quite as annoyed had he been asked the question during the daytime rather than in the middle of the night. Indeed, you could ask why the question could not wait until the next day. (By the way, some doctors do not function very well when woken during the night. I think it was sleep-induced automatic behaviour that led another friend to respond to the mid-night plea from the nurse, "Mr. Smith is having difficulty sleeping" with the response "So am I!")

The concept of taking a treatment regularly and quite possibly permanently tends not to go down well with people. It is easy to feel that you are giving out a life sentence, rather than possibly a lifesaving treatment, when telling someone that they will have to take this medication for the rest of their life. As one patient put it, "Forever!!! Do you mean for the rest of my life?" I felt like saying, "Well, not afterwards" but, as usual, refrained.

A patient's response is usually followed by the question "But what are the side effects?" This is a perfectly reasonable question because most drugs have side effects although fortunately not in most people; otherwise, they would never get onto the market. Some side effects and the circumstances of their discovery and management are, however, dramatic.

Poisons and medicine are oftentimes the same substance given with different intents. Peter Mere Latham

The trendsetter in severe side effects was thalidomide, which was introduced in the 1950s as a sedative but was also found to be effective in the alleviation of morning sickness in pregnancy. Consequently, it was widely prescribed to pregnant women, except in the United States where it was not licensed. Although it was probably believed at the time that drugs could not cross the placenta to reach and damage the developing child, these ideas rapidly changed when the drug was found to be responsible for numerous birth defects, including phocomelia, a condition in which the newborn's limbs are typically underdeveloped and deformed with stunting and missing sections. Thalidomide was probably responsible for about ten thousand cases of phocomelia.

The drug was withdrawn in the United Kingdom in 1961 and regulations concerning the testing and licensing of new medicines were considerably tightened. Did that prevent future disasters? Unfortunately not.

Mr. Jack Ashley, MP for Stoke-on-Trent South, spoke about the anti-arthritis drug, Opren, in the House of Commons in 1983. He described a dramatic collapse of confidence in the drug after "a meteoric rise in popularity" seemingly because the drug was responsible for nearly three thousand reports of adverse reaction, including seventy-six deaths. Enough to make anyone or anything unpopular, some would say. Salt was rubbed into the wound, according to Mr. Ashley (although he didn't actually put it that way) by the parent company which was accused of deliberately concealing the adverse reactions.

Psaty and colleagues wrote in the Journal of the American Medical Association in 2004 about the drug cerivastatin, which was launched onto the market in 1998 as treatment to reduce levels of cholesterol in the blood. They concluded that the drug's serious side effects included destruction of muscle tissue and kidney failure. Importantly, the risk was much higher with cerivastatin than with other similar drugs that lower blood cholesterol. Psaty and his friends said that the Company's own documents suggested a problem with the drug within approximately one hundred days of the launch on to the market in 1998 but a warning was not added to the package insert for more than eighteen months. Other findings by the Company itself that the risk of muscle destruction with cerivastatin was greater than with a similar drug were not "to our knowledge" disseminated or published, they add. Cerivastatin was removed from the market in August 2001.

They conclude "Despite limitations of the available data, the asymmetry between the information available to the Company and the information available to patients and physicians seems striking", a remark which no doubt terminated the authors' participation in the Company's dinner party circuit.

The Daily Mirror of Nov 21, 2002 included an article that stated the following: "A miracle drug intended to stop epileptic seizures has instead wrecked the lives of many. One victim tells her shocking story. By Jill Palmer"

"After years of suffering debilitating seizures Janette Whitehead was delighted with a revolutionary new drug."

"Vigabatrin (Sabril) was hailed as a major breakthrough in the treatment of epilepsy. It was the first new drug for 10 years and highly successful in reducing and even stopping seizures."

"But tragically the drug she took to improve her life has virtually ruined it."

"It has severely damaged her eyes, leaving Janette with tunnel vision and partially sighted."

"Now she has joined 30 other victims in legal action against the manufacturer Aventis Pharma. 'The drug that was meant to make my life easier has made it even harder' said Janette, 46, from Totnes, South Devon."

This serious side effect, which can lead to virtually complete blindness, occurs in thirty percent or more of patients taking the drug. The damage to vision is irreversible.

Half the modern drugs could well be thrown out the window, except that the birds might eat them. Martin H. Fischer

The Sun of 19 September 2004 stated: "The parents of a nine-year-old boy are suing the makers of an epilepsy drug that may have caused their son to go blind. Carl and Pamela Beedle have launched a legal action against the makers of vigabatrin, which son Ryan has taken since he was just months old."

"The couple are one of 200 families involved in the High Court claim, which could result in millions of pounds in compensation being paid. Stephen Hanbury, of Wolferstans Solicitors in Plymouth, who are handling the claims against Aventis Pharma, said: 'Although there are warnings about the drug now, there weren't any at the time when Ryan started taking the drug.'"

An internet forum in 2006 contained the following comments:

"This class action has been very quiet since it was launched since (*sic*) early 2000."

"Most likely a settlement has been reached out of court, and all who were involved were given payment, told not to stir the pot, or they themselves would be sued."

"What you say about the case being settled out of court and the plaintiffs paid off with hush money is very probably true and more than sad."

Needless to say, none of these reported allegations against the pharmaceutical industry is necessarily true.

Confusion over the facts may sometimes come from other sources. The drug Debendox (also known as Bendectin in some countries) was introduced in 1956 as treatment for nausea in pregnancy. Like thalidomide, it became implicated in the cause of birth defects and numerous law suits followed. The manufacturer voluntarily withdrew the drug from the market in 1983. One of the experts involved in the claims against Debendox was Dr. McBride who alerted the world to the dangers of thalidomide.

The Independent published an article on 20 February 1993 which reported that Dr. McBride had been found guilty of scientific fraud over his experiments with Debendox.

The article said that the Medical Tribunal of New South Wales accused Dr. McBride of "deliberately selecting and culling data" and of "reprehensible" conduct in his experiments. It described the affair as "a sorry saga" which should have been avoided.

Later on, the article states that Dr. McBride admitted to the medical tribunal that he had altered data about drug dosages given to rabbits and had taken short cuts which a scientist should not take. As a result, he had published material which was false and misleading. Dr. McBride apparently regretted all this.

According to the Independent, he privately asserted that big international drug companies were behind his downfall and that he was a victim of a conspiracy. He apparently once said, "It's all very well to talk about perfect scientific protocol. Drug companies have a vested interest in keeping their drugs on the market. I have a vested interest in protecting unborn babies. It's as simple as that."

Which side of this argument makes a representation closer to the truth is, of course, unclear but one thing is certain - articles like that do not help the subject of the story to get research grants.

But I can't think for you. You'll have to decide. Bob Dylan "With God on our Side"

Fortunately, despite possible failings of industry and the medical profession, many medical conditions have been transformed for the better by new drugs, which all goes to show that you can still make a good apple pie from class II apples.

Many drugs can cause people to become a bit muddle-headed, or to fall asleep in polite company, but some have much more remarkable effects on behaviour. One treatment for Parkinson's disease is a class of drugs known as dopamine agonists, which includes medicines with names such as ropinirole, pramipexole and cabergoline. From around 2000, doctors began to recognise that all was not well in the lives of some people taking these treatments. In retrospect, it was probably rather easy to identify the changes as drug side effects because they were a bit more dramatic than your average headache and included uncontrolled gambling and shopping, pathological jealousy and becoming frankly oversexed (although not necessarily all at the same time).

James Allen was a sixty-eight-year-old man who had had Parkinson's disease for eight years. At one of his outpatient visits, he reported that his existing treatment seemed not to be working so well because there were times during the day when he had a great deal of difficulty in walking and using his hands but others when everything seemed fine. Recognising that this fluctuation in symptoms during a single day is one of the complications of Parkinson's disease, my registrar suggested adding cabergoline, one of the dopamine agonist drugs, to his existing medication and I agreed. We started him on a low dose, gave him instructions how to increase the dose gradually over the next three weeks and arranged to see him again in the outpatient clinic four weeks later.

One week before his scheduled appointment, his general practitioner telephoned to tell me that Mrs. Allen was at her wits end because her usually calm and long-suffering husband was convinced that she was having an affair and had become so distraught at this belief that he spent hours repeatedly searching through her belongings and studying the numbers listed on their itemised telephone bill for evidence of her misdemeanours. He virtually refused to let her out of the house for fear that her lover might be waiting around the corner. Even her carrying large bags of shopping back to the house when she did manage to break free failed to convince him of her innocent (and rather unexciting motives) for leaving the house because she was clearly capable of accommodating a sexual encounter during her shopping trip to Tesco, even if she went on the bus. Probably contrary to most people's experience, Mr. Allen was of the view that supermarkets are rarely so crowded as to prevent the practice of clandestine sex somewhere between the tropical fruit juice and the spray-on deodorants (adding a whole new meaning to the phrase "processed meat", I felt). The critical piece of evidence in support of his theory, he later explained, was the finding of his wife's underwear in the boot of the family car. He admitted on enquiry that the circumstances that had led to this phenomenon defied a simple explanation and he could only speculate how the frillies had ended up as next-door neighbours to the spare wheel.

At this point, I was reminded of a story related to me by a consultant psychiatrist when I was a student. Dr. Langston was trying to teach us about delusions, which form part of some psychiatric disorders, such as schizophrenia. A delusion, he explained, is a false belief strongly held despite overwhelming evidence to the contrary. One of the patients in the secure (i.e. locked) ward at a famous psychiatric hospital had schizophrenia and had claimed relentlessly since his admission two years earlier that he was a personal friend of the Archbishop of York, despite having the appearance of a down-and-out hobo. This belief was recorded as one of his fixed delusions until, one day, the Archbishop came unannounced to visit him, having learned that his old friend had become ill. Because the criterion of "despite overwhelming evidence to the contrary" was not fulfilled, explained Dr. Langston, the definition of the belief as a delusion was no longer appropriate. I suppose you could argue that the prejudice of the psychiatric team when assessing the man's initial claims was also inappropriate.

Not wishing to make a similar mistake with Mr. Allen, I felt compelled to determine as far as possible whether or not his belief was true. Thus I questioned Mrs. Allen quite frankly but stopped short of eliciting her theories as to how her underwear could possibly have found its way into the boot of the car. She quite simply denied categorically that she was having an affair and pointed out that her husband's current behaviour was abnormal regardless of any other consideration because, by contrast, he had reacted with singular indifference when he found out about her real affair fifteen years earlier.

We admitted Mr. Allen to hospital and gradually withdrew the cabergoline treatment. Three days after completely stopping the drug, he seemed a lot less agitated.

"How are you, Mr. Allen?" I enquired on the ward round.

"Fine."

"You seem to be a lot calmer. Do you still think your wife is having an affair?" I asked.

"I do, actually," he replied "but I'm not bothered about it any more."

Anybody who cannot cope with uncertain situations, unanswered questions or imperfect outcomes should not go into medicine.

The Telegraph, on 28 October 2009, described a fifty-nine-year-old man who worked as a £50,000 per year IT manager before retiring. He claimed "that after he was prescribed cabergoline seven years ago his personality completely changed."

"He....started spending money on a high life, handing over £400,000..... and hiring Bentleys, Ferraris and classic Jaguar cars."

"He ran up.....debts on 15 credit cards, became violent to his second wife and started wearing women's frilly underwear after developing a cross-dressing habit."

"Hull Crown Court heard that this led him to carrying out a ticket scam, selling tickets for Take That and Donny Osmond that didn't actually exist over eBay."

"He carried out the ruse over an 11-month period from 2007 during which time 172 people paid £45,718 for tickets they never received."

Following medical advice, the judge gave him a conditional discharge because his responsibility for what he did was "very substantially" reduced by the side effects of the drug.

The article also reported a former headmaster who received an absolute discharge the previous year after a judge at Oxford Crown Court ruled that the Parkinson's disease drugs cabergoline and ropinirole were responsible for his amassing thousands of indecent images of children.

It is amazing and disturbing that a drug, of a pefectly legal kind, can almost commit its user to a life behind bars.

Thalidomide, Opren, cerivastatin, vigabatrin and the dopamine agonist drugs have two things in common. The first is that they are all very effective treatments in their respective fields so there is a strong impetus to prescribe them. The second is that the conditions that result as serious drug side effects occur naturally, without drugs, very rarely so a spurt of cases over a few years is very easily spotted as related to use of a particular medication. What might reasonably keep us awake at night with worry is the drug that is not prescribed very often and which, as a side effect, increases the risk of something common, such as bowel cancer. A lot of cases would have to occur before the link to the drug was suspected. But not to increase amongst my readers the paranoia that currently exists about the dangers of prescription drugs in the general population, I should point out that drugs could equally have a *benefit* that is so far undetected - who knows, your hay fever spray may stop you getting prostate cancer.

Some drugs, including the dopamine agonists used in Parkinson's disease, commonly produce hallucinations whereby people see things that are not actually there. Consultants who run Parkinson's disease clinics become very used to their patients' letting them know about the wasps that fly through their hands "amazingly without causing any pain or indeed any sensation at all", the ants crawling over the carpet, walls and furniture and the people who turn up in the lounge without invitation, who refuse to speak and who ignore requests, polite or otherwise, to leave. Because these visions appear very real to those who experience them, there is rarely any point in arguing about their veracity for fear of implying to the patient that he or she is a downright liar or a candidate for the locked ward at the nearest psychiatric hospital. Some hallucinations are distressing but others are just a nuisance.

Mrs. Bradbury's were rather special. She had been taking cabergoline for Parkinson's disease for some years without side effects but, at a recent outpatient visit, we increased the dose quite substantially because she could not get about as well as she used to do. She returned to her scheduled appointment two months later.

"How are you, Mrs. Bradbury?" I enquired. "Has the increase in the cabergoline had any effect?"

"Oh yes," she replied. "I can get about much better."

"Have you had any side effects?"

"No," she said a little hesitatingly. "The only strange thing is that every night that I get into bed, a man comes and lies down beside me."

Mrs. Bradbury was widowed and, as far as I knew, had not acquired any suitors recently. She also told me that the occurrence was strange, which I decided was not the adjective she would have chosen to describe any new relationship taken on voluntarily. I could not imagine that a woman of her demeanour and age would engage in any "strange" bedtime practices. The experiences must have been hallucinations.

"Do you believe that it is really happening, that a man is truly getting into bed with you?" I asked.

"Well, not if I think about it but it does seem very real."

Her hallucinations were not so severe as to cause total loss of insight and I was able to explain that the cabergoline was likely to be the culprit and that we had better cut back the dose and try some other treatment instead in case the side effects became more severe and she started having visions that were very frightening for her. She agreed.

Two weeks later she came back to the clinic as planned.

"How are you now?" I asked. "Is the new treatment as effective as the cabergoline was?"

"Yes, I am pleased to say that I have not really noticed any difference. I am still able to do as much as I was on the cabergoline."

"Any new side-effects?"

"No, fortunately," she replied.

"And the night-time experiences - is a man still coming to lie beside you in bed?"

"No, unfortunately."

Because drugs are an integral part of treatment for a physician, most consultants have at least some involvement with the pharmaceutical industry. Some doctors, it is true, refuse to have contact with anybody who has ever been found within one hundred yards of a drug company's premises for fear that their pure, open minds may be sullied by the obvious gross bias of the company representative. Personally, I have always found it a little depressing that such senior doctors admit to being so gullible.

Most doctors are prepared to boast a greater degree of intellectual resistance and engage in some form of working relationship with the guys who make the pills. The benefits are mutual: the company hopes to have their product prescribed (i.e sold) and to receive advice and assistance from someone who might know at least as much as they do about the condition; the doctor receives goods, facilities and money that range through company-monogrammed sticky pads, provision of advisory services to doctors and patients, payment for drug trials and sponsorship for attendance at and participation in conferences. There is also a certain kudos, real or imagined, in being a member of an advisory committee to a major pharmaceutical company and it does no harm to a CV that may be under consideration for a merit award.

Most drug company executives know very well how to tap into the consultant's sense of self-importance and willingly offer appropriate baits to gain their side of the bargain. For several years, I was a member of a particular advisory committee that existed, as far as I could judge, in an entirely virtual and inert form because there were never any meetings and I do not recall ever advising substantially on anything. It did, however, allow the company executive to telephone me at regular intervals "to touch base" or, more precisely, to remind me of the existence of him, his company and his product and to let me know the latest piece of evidence to prove that his drug remained superior to all competitors.

I like to think that there is at least an element of altruism on the part of the pharmaceutical industry in sponsoring doctors to attend conferences because these meetings are mostly educational and many medics would not be able to afford to go or at least would be unwilling to spend their own money on an activity that does not work out cheap. If the commercial financial support requires its recipient to give a talk in a special session devoted to an area of medicine dear to the company's heart, because it happens to have a drug for use in that area, it is almost possible to convince oneself that one is simply being paid in kind for services rendered. Admittedly, it would be a fairly good rate of reimbursement - five nights in a four-star hotel in some exotic place, coverage of the conference registration fee and dinner in a different restaurant every evening is a good rate of return for a twenty-minute talk with slides.

.....people talk of situations, read books, repeat quotations, draw conclusions on the wall. Bob Dylan "Love Minus Zero/No Limit"

Maybe occasionally the game is overplayed. In the Parliamentary sitting on 27 January 1983, Mr. Jack Ashley made reference to recent television programmes on the arthritis drug Opren. He said "'Panorama' did two splendid programmes on Opren and revealed a disturbing picture of the relationship between drug companies and the medical profession. If 'Panorama' is right, there is no doubt that some people in the medical profession are bribed by the drug companies."

David Crouch, MP for Canterbury, stated that a drug company had taken "the Orient Express to Venice to talk to doctors, rather than talking to them in Manchester—as I think one of the doctors said could have been done, although he added, with a smile, 'I don't think that I would have gone to Manchester, rather than to Venice.' Even so, it stretches my credulity to think that a junket on the Orient Express is the way to promote an idea among rheumatology consultants. It is a pity." Oh dear! Not my experience, I have to say.

Sometimes I get the feeling the aspirin companies are sponsoring my headaches.   Terri Guillemets

All in all, for most people, working with the pharmaceutical industry is a pleasant experience. Participation in drug trials really does help to produce new medicines because, without those trials, the drugs could never be licensed. It also allows the consultant to feel important. Involvement on advisory committees can sometimes be useful. I remember once pointing out to the company team that the proposed packaging for capsules to treat patients with Parkinson's disease, who usually have manipulative difficulties, was inappropriate because no representative of the human race would be capable of releasing the pills from their sealed plastic wrapper without some form of specialised industrial cutting equipment and the Parkinson's patients would be barred from using the equipment on health and safety grounds. (It was, of course, important to include the reference to Parkinson's disease in my statement because otherwise the advice could easily have been given by a non-neurologist or even a non-medic, a situation that would have destroyed my indispensability and thus one not to be desired.)

The trips to conferences abroad were mostly exciting, at least during early experiences, and even allowed time to learn something new in an otherwise busy programme of sight-seeing, dining and learning how to handle speedboats. Being accommodated in a converted Italian monastery, free of charge, in a marble-floored suite of rooms with a total area greater than the average New York apartment, walls decorated with original frescos and lullabies provided by nightingales was arguably a unique experience for anyone except the original monks.

After a while, it is true, the trips can become not so rosy. Repetitive air flights to distant lands and staying in hotels, however many stars they have, can be tedious as many business people will testify. (There is also only a limited number of converted Italian monasteries.) And you never know who you are going to find yourself next to at dinner - sometimes interesting, sometimes fun, sometimes exciting and sometimes downright boring. A heavy dose of the sedative that is red or white, comes in seventy-five centilitre bottles and is served in stemmed glasses is often required to protect the sensorium from the sustained onslaught of one's neighbour in giving his current views on the best way to manage stroke in the rural districts of Cumberland.

But it all passes the time between patients.

On a sunny morning following my return from an arduous conference in Florida, the fatigue from which had been eased only by travel in the business class section of the aircraft with its king-size chairbeds and hand-served claret, I received a request from a general practitioner to see one of his patients urgently. The young man in question (he was twenty-one) had collapsed unconscious outside his front door as he was about to put his key into the lock. A neighbour, who happened to be returning home about the same time, witnessed the event and called an ambulance which travelled urgently to the scene. By the time of its arrival, the man was beginning to come round. Unfortunately, the caring attention from the paramedic, who tried to move him into the recovery position to prevent choking, was rewarded by a punch on the nose from his newly acquired patient.

When all the dust had settled, and the bleeding from the paramedic's nose had been stemmed, it was established by all fourteen of the neighbours who had torn themselves away from Coronation Street to investigate the furore outside their windows, that the seemingly aggressive outburst by the young man whom they knew as Wayne was quite atypical. He was unlikely to be drunk or otherwise intoxicated because his life to date had been unsullied by use of the mind-bending chemicals relied upon by so many inferiors of his generation. He was much more likely to be found looking after the hamsters that he produced from his part-time semi-commercial breeding programme. As far as they knew, of course.

The young man corroborated the blameless nature of the lifestyle recounted by his neighbours, adding by way of confirmation that sales of hamsters had increased this year by thirty percent compared with the previous year. He had no idea why he had smacked the paramedic and furthermore couldn't remember doing it.

The neighbour who had been first on the scene offered the suggestion that Wayne had had some sort of fit apparently based on the evidence that "it looked as if he was having some sort of fit". On more detailed enquiry, it turned out that he had seen Wayne go stiff in the arms and legs and then start to jerk rhythmically whilst lying on the floor.

Wayne reported that he had never had any attacks like this before. I agreed with the general practitioner that he had probably had his first epileptic attack and that he required further investigation. The aggressive behaviour that led to the misfortune of the paramedic in attendance was part of a confusional state that often follows major epileptic attacks. It was not done deliberately or indeed with any real awareness by Wayne of what he was doing which is why he could remember nothing about it afterwards. None of this was particularly unusual.

A few weeks later, I received a letter from a firm of solicitors which informed me that they were representing a certain Wayne Thompson who had been charged with assault and was due to appear in court. They told me that he had collapsed outside his home. When a paramedic came to look after him, Mr. Thompson allegedly forcibly and deliberately struck the paramedic in the region of the centre of his face, thereby occasioning nasal trauma and consequent bleeding. The defence was that Mr. Thompson had no memory of the assault or indeed of the arrival of the paramedic. The lawyers required an opinion on whether the blackout, assault and loss of memory were related and whether they were due to a neurological disorder.

It struck me as a remarkable coincidence if there were two Waynes, each of whom had suffered a blackout outside their home, struck a paramedic and had no memory for it afterwards (although, on reflection, I realised that Wayne was quite a common name and, for all I knew, the other features of the coincidence may all be quite frequent events in Hillsborough). A brief scan of my notes relating to the first case confirmed that the two Waynes were indeed one and the same. It was then quite easy to produce a report that confirmed, from a medical standpoint, the legal defence of Wayne Thompson.

With this one case, I found myself entering another arena that was unsuspected at the start of medical studies or through most of my training: The Law. Henceforeward I was to have regular brushes with police, solicitors, barristers and judges without once being convicted. I don't remember my Teddy bear warning me about this.

Chapter 10: Legal requirements

If there were no bad people, there would be no good lawyers. Charles Dickens

These days, someone injured in an accident is as likely to be looked after by a lawyer as a doctor.

"Dr. Sagar, do come in," said the man in the pinstripe suit. "I am Charles Spencer, Prosecution Counsel in this case and here are Tom Jenkins and Victoria Gleeson from the Crown Prosecution Service. Thank you very much for coming at such short notice. Do take a seat. Can I offer you tea, coffee, water? Please help yourself and I will explain our quandary." I was about to embark on my first substantive medicolegal experience.

Charles Spencer was a decidedly portly gentleman with jowls that just overflowed onto his starched collar. His face bordered on an unhealthy shade of red and his eyebrows curled outwards at the edges. Most of the time, his face was fixed in an immobile mask with dark penetrating eyes that looked out from under his hirsute eyebrows. His voice was resonant and pronunciation precise but slightly clipped. His whole persona resembled that of John Mortimer's Rumpole of the Bailey.

"Jason Blackheath, aged thirty-six years, is currently on trial for the murder of his next-door neighbour, a certain

Dale Avery, who was fatally wounded with a knife around 6 p.m. on 14 April 1984" he explained.

"Part of the way through the trial, somewhat belatedly in my view," he expanded, with a sideways glance at his colleagues from the CPS, both of whom were staring at the ground "we learn that the accused has longstanding epilepsy. A key feature of his defence is that he has no memory of the assault. I should add that identification of our friend Mr. Blackheath as the perpetrator of the fatal wounding is beyond reasonable doubt for various reasons, most of which I will not relate in order not to bore you, save that he was caught by another neighbour at the scene of the fatal wounding with the knife in his hand, all of this having been recorded on said neighbour's camera, which is maintained on his person at all times, pending the need to produce a photographic record in the event of damages inflicted by another, accidentally or purposefully, upon his person or property." One seldom finds people capable of speaking long sentences without sounding more than faintly ridiculous but lawyers are foremost amongst them.

It is the trade of lawyers to question everything, yield nothing, and talk by the hour. Thomas Jefferson

He continued: "The question has been raised, and it is on this that I require your expert opinion, as to whether the accused could have been in some form of epileptic seizure that led not only to his unwittingly inflicting fatal wounds to Mr.

Avery's body but also to having no memory of having done so afterwards because, if so, our friend Mr. Blackheath could, or at least in principle could, successfully plead a defence of automatism which, in this situation, would more likely than not lead to his acquittal, an outcome sought, of course, with ardour by our defence colleagues but one which, for us, would be quite disappointing, not least because we believe him to be guilty."

"Why in particular do you believe him to be guilty?" I asked.

"For a number of reasons but principally three. First, this defence only surfaced once the trial had begun; it does not appear in his witness statement. Second, he had been free of epileptic seizures for ten years before this incident and, third, because he stated to police in interview that his neighbour 'had it coming to him.'"

I explained that some forms of epileptic seizure can indeed lead to involuntary behaviour, including violence, and loss of memory for the period of the seizure. However, the attacks come on suddenly and without reason.

After some further years of medicolegal experience, I learnt that barristers usually know the answers to questions before they ask them and that their pleas of ignorance of medical matters usually shield an encyclopaedic knowledge that could probably fit them in no time with a medical degree if they bothered to pursue it. But it obviously helps to keep the dagger in the cloak.

"It may help you, Dr. Sagar", he went on, "if I were to explain some of the circumstances of the case, in light of your latter comments concerning the characteristics of automatic behaviour and amnesia in epileptic seizures, for which, by the way, I am grateful."

"It transpires – and all the witnesses agree on this – that Avery, the victim, nurtured a longstanding affair with Blackheath's wife. The meetings were clandestine and conducted while Blackheath was at work. Avery's unique – as far as this case is concerned, that is – unique work pattern characterised by shifts doubtless facilitated the secretive liaisons because Avery was often at home during the day whereas Blackheath did not benefit from this working arrangement. Unfortunately, as all too often happens it seems, Blackheath returned home unexpectedly at around 2 p.m. one day to find Avery in a state of flagrante delicto with his wife – Blackheath's, that is. A row ensued, perhaps not surprisingly, but on this occasion Mrs. Blackheath achieved success in calming the would-be-combatants."

"The following day, to cut a long story short, Avery returned home and was about to enter his domicile by the front entrance when Blackheath, who apparently was waiting in his car, ran up the drive of Avery and stabbed him in the back with a knife later identified by Mrs. Blackheath – and incidentally confirmed by Mr. Blackheath - as being one of their domestic carving knives. Indeed, later forensic examination confirmed the weapon as being one of a set of similar knives possessed by the Blackheaths."

"When Blackheath was asked how the knife came to be in his motor vehicle, no explanation was forthcoming. Mrs. Blackheath's evidence, should the Court care to accept it – and I would be the first to submit that there may be good reasons for not so doing – is that Mr. Blackheath had not returned home since leaving that morning, a conclusion about which she can be particularly confident because infirmity in their pet cat had caused her to remain indoors for the whole of the daylight hours. The logical conclusion from Mrs. Blackheath's evidence is that the knife left the domicile in the morning with Mr. Blackheath, most probably carried by him from the house to the car, where it remained until fulfilling its grizzly purpose later in the day."

I indicated that the clear elements of premeditation involved in the attack were not features of epileptic automatism which therefore was unlikely to be a reliable explanation of an unfortunate sequence of events.

"Certainly unfortunate for Mr. Avery, Dr. Sagar," said Charles Spencer, "and, in light of your comments, quite possibly also for Mr. Blackheath once the trial has concluded. I am grateful to you. I believe you have confirmed to my colleagues in the Crown Prosecution Service your willingness to give evidence in court should you be so required."

"Yes, indeed. Can I just make one comment?"

"Yes, of course," effused Charles. "Please go ahead." Barristers can be so polite.

"I may be being naive but isn't loss of memory put forward quite often as defence in criminal law?"

Charles seemed to inflate in front of my eyes. His chest and abdomen expanded; he drew himself back in his chair; and the facial hue shifted several degrees from its position of borderline healthy red to one well within the clearly unhealthy range.

"Dr. Sagar," he began with the tone and volume of a Shakespearian soliloquy "you would be amazed just how often, when the murder weapon is about to enter the body, down comes this big blue cloud and erases all memory of the event."

Barristers ride words like surfers ride waves.

The activities that lure a consultant away from arguably a primary role in caring for patients that, Dear Reader, you have heard about so far include management, research and generation of professional warfare. To that list, we must add medico-legal work which involves providing advice to lawyers dealing with cases concerning medical matters. The consultant is acting in a capacity of an "expert witness" although quite who decides on the expert qualification is usually unclear. Ultimately, it is the lawyer seeking the opinion but usually the expert is chosen from a group of individuals whose characteristics in common include the willingness to be classed as expert. Thus, as in any field, important jobs are effectively often held by self-appointees.

Medics deal with legal cases in three categories: personal injury, medical negligence and criminal law. Most of the personal injury cases concern compensation for injury acquired in an accident, usually motor-vehicle or work-related. In neurology, the commonest problem is head injury, the effects of which vary according to severity from minor headache and dizziness to permanent brain damage and loss of independent living. The negligence cases concern neurological injury caused by unreasonable medical care. Neurological input into criminal cases is required when the accused may have a defence or is not fit to stand trial because of some neurological disorder.

A neurologist would also have the expertise to advise on how to mimic a neurological condition to avoid trial or to fake a compensation claim but so far I have had no requests for these services, which I believe are illegal. I did once have to advise an actress on how to portray a patient with multiple sclerosis but I think she was a bona fide participant in a commercial production and, at that time at least, involved in no legal claim. (It does make you think, though, that the information I gave would set her up for a fake claim in the future, if she so chose.)

Because there is a cash reward at stake, compensation claims can attract the fraudster, not the professional who specialises in duplication of the rest of the world's credit cards and passports but the amateur who sees pound signs whenever he or she experiences any kind of medical discomfort. All physical problems have psychological components. Chronic pain, for example, may produce depression which itself makes the pain harder to bear and therefore worse as far as the sufferer is concerned. This psychological process is subconscious. On the other side of the coin is the conscious fabrication, or malingering, for effect. Unfortunately, the two often coexist or metamorphose each into the other. The genuine disability following an accident may recover but it may suit the claimant to pretend that it continues because, that way, they do not have to return to work and moreover in English law will be paid for the privilege.

A lot of time is spent in argument between the two sides of the compensation claim with one legal team, strangely always the claimant's, arguing vociferously that it is staggering that their client can even breathe, let alone work and the other, equally strangely always the defendant's, pointing out that the accident victim could be a pentathlon champion if only they put their mind to it and stopped pretending otherwise. To be fair to the defendant's team, they do usually stop short of arguing that the accident has serendipitously *improved* the claimant's abilities.

The two sides are always backed up by medical expertise because the lawyers have years of experience in identifying which consultant is most likely to back their case. Hawks and Doves feature as much in doctors' personalities as anywhere else. The canniest lawyers, however, know that consultants easily gain a reputation for bias, particularly if it is always in favour of the fee payer so choose experts who will tend to favour the claimant or defendant's side within a generally balanced opinion. Left of centre or right of centre is much preferable to communist or fascist in this situation.

If an expert says it can't be done, get another expert.
David Ben-Gurion

Compensation is directly related to the financial principle of restoring the life of the injured party to what it would have been had the disabling event never occurred. Because the financial rewards are greater the less an individual is able to do, a whole army of surveillance experts has spawned with the prime aim of proving that the affected person is able to do more than they claim. Strangely, these services are always recruited by the defendant's side, usually the insurance company or its lawyers. The surveillance team covertly follows the claimant, filming their every move, over a period of sometimes several days and then presents their findings on a CD, where the footage is accompanied by a voiceover explaining the circumstances. Unfortunately, since most claimants are broadly telling the truth, the recorded physical activities tend to be rather meagre.

I have spent many happy hours watching videos of the front doors of houses, which we are reliably informed by the voiceover, is the "domicile of the subject", enlivened from time to time by a face passing a front window. Excitement mounts when we see Subject leave the house and travel as a passenger in a car to the local supermarket, returning to the car after twenty to thirty minutes and travelling back home, maybe carrying one bag. Another common "on location" feature is a person, just about recognisable as the claimant, walking down the street. Much is made of these recordings: "Your client claims not to be able to walk for more than fifteen minutes without discomfort but the surveillance video shows him walking without difficulty." A major flaw in the argument is that the recording of the walking person ceases after just ten minutes.

I have certainly seen more interesting videos than the surveillance ones but I cannot imagine how my boredom in watching them compares with that of the people recording them. I am reminded of the film "Sleep" by Andy Warhol (1963) that records someone asleep for about six hours. Perhaps the surveillance company sees their product as a similar art form.

Maybe also the excitement of the ultimate catch outweighs all the tedium of waiting. The catch can certainly be dramatic, the thirty-four-pound salmon that makes the day standing in the River Tay all worthwhile. A thirty-year-old man was said to be paralysed from the waist down after a road accident and confined to a wheelchair. Everyone, lawyers and medics alike, seemed convinced – until the video landed on the front door mat of the claimant's lawyers. The man was filmed driving to a consultant's practice rooms for an assessment, accompanied by a male passenger in the front seat. On arrival, the claimant got out of the car, walked to the boot and lifted out a wheelchair in which he sat. His friend pushed him to the consultation. Afterwards the procedure was repeated in reverse order.

Another star video featured a twenty-eight-year-old man who allegedly had a useless right arm due to nerve damage acquired in an operation on his armpit. The producers of this epic left no stones unturned in their efforts to generate audience-gripping action. The expense involved in spraying all the cars in the street with mud was justified at the moment that they filmed the fulfilment of their prediction: the man vigorously washing his car using both arms. Gotcha!

Cases such as these collapse instantly but they are rare. Most of the output of the surveillance film industry features long studies of people doing not very much.

Recognition of a medical condition as a cause of altered, even illegal, behaviour is relatively new but astute criminal lawyers now jump for the telephone at the first discovery that their client has a medical disorder in order to seek expert opinion on a possible defence.

As a budding doctor and later budding consultant, I never dreamt that my professional activities would include rape (as an advisor, that is, not the perpetrator). But a letter of instruction from the defence solicitors informed me that Martin Clough, aged twenty, was due to stand trial for the rape of an eighteen-year-old girl whose identity was withheld for her protection (unlike him). The complication was that, two hours before, he had sustained a minor head injury and the issue at stake was whether this could have caused him unwittingly to rape the girl. My first reaction was that, if so, it is surprising that rape had not been inflicted on at least ninety percent of the female population of inner cities given the frequency of minor head injury in alcohol and testosterone-fuelled young men when the pubs close. However, as usual, I kept the thoughts to myself and agreed to consider the case.

It turned out that Martin had had a certain contretemps with a fellow imbiber at a public house near the Northern General Hospital and had lost out in the duel outside that followed. A swift right hook had knocked him to the ground and caused his head to strike a wheelie bin on the way down. The wheelie bin apparently sustained no ill effects but Martin was rendered unconscious for a few minutes. On coming round, he had a headache and dizziness and felt sick so he decided to walk home rather than move on to a late night drinking establishment for more sustenance.

By the time he had got to the bus stop on Hucklow Road, twenty minutes later, he was feeling much better. It was then that he encountered Miss Anonymous (who by then I knew to be a certain Tracey Mills), the girlfriend of one of his mates, waiting at the bus stop. According to the prosecution, he dragged Miss Mills into the darker recesses of Firth Park where he became sexually gratified at her expense and without her consent. According to Martin, they were both highly aroused sexually at the mere sight of each other and took things on to the next logical step.

There was not much chance of getting him off using the defence of automatism – committing the attack without any voluntary control – because he could recall all the details well and moreover said the act was consensual. Unless he was so deluded by the effects of the head injury as to imagine that an act of rape was in fact carried out with her agreement, I could offer no medical explanation for his conduct. Furthermore, if he were so deluded, the head injury would probably have been more severe and he would not have remembered everything so well. Despite my misgivings, the defence barrister asked me to attend the trial in case anything came up in evidence that might be medically relevant.

In cross-examination, he asked young Tracey how she had come to report the crime and she explained that she did so at her boyfriend's assistance when she told him that rape was the explanation of why she and Martin had been seen together near the park that evening. They were seen by a mutual friend who, with everyone's welfare presumably as his prime concern, had passed on the information to Tracey's boyfriend. It was no doubt pure coincidence that Tracey had dumped the well-wisher for her new boyfriend three months earlier.

Tracey admitted in cross-examination Martin's claim that he interrupted the intercourse in order to pass water and that she requested removal of her tights because they were tightening around her legs during the rape. She also admitted that Martin temporarily ceased his sexual assault to allow her to carry out this partial *deshabillement* and resumed once she had completed it. She didn't really know why she had not run away when he left her to use a nearby tree as a urinal. When Defence Counsel pointed out that Well-Wisher had seen them walking together peacefully towards the park, she indicated that she had walked back to the scene of the crime, accompanied by the alleged rapist, ten minutes later because she had forgotten her tights.

Martin didn't need me. The Jury found him unanimously not guilty.

It may be true that the law cannot make a man love me, but it can keep him from lynching me, and I think that's pretty important. Martin Luther King Jr

The jury consist of twelve persons chosen to decide who has the better lawyer. Robert Frost

Getting to see the accused in a pending criminal trial can be tricky to organise, not least because the client is usually in prison on remand. Life in medicine is a series of surprises. Until having spent several years as a consultant, I would never have dreamt that one day I would have had so much time inside that I could have been a tour guide to the best of Britain's prisons. I can assure most prisoners that getting into a prison is probably not much easier than getting out. Making the appointment with the prison services is the easy bit but what follows thereafter is a series of blocks to stumble the unwary and prevent the fulfilment of the objective.

First is the negotiation with the greeting party on the reception desk. I know they have been trained correctly to maintain security but it is nevertheless quite unnerving to be labelled by default as an escaped prisoner/importer into the prison of drugs, weapons or other undesirables/dodgy solicitor until proven otherwise. The appointment so carefully arranged in advance seems never to appear on the prison's written agenda for the day. However, being only too willing to help, the staff on reception are often prepared to undertake a telephone call to establish one's permission to exist.

Unfortunately, one call seldom suffices; by the time the arrangements have been confirmed, a whole series of calls appears to have been made in order to find out who exactly is responsible for the arrival on their doorstep of this vagrant, disguised in a suit and tie and carrying a briefcase. I can only imagine it culminates in a chat with HM Governor of Prisons.

On one of these occasions, I was reminded of an event at the Radcliffe Infirmary in Oxford some years previously. Late one evening, long after the sun had gone to bed, the night porter on duty observed a man walking down the corridor with a moderate stoop and a slight stagger. On looking more closely, he noticed that the man was wearing a medical white coat but other semblances to professionalism were largely absent. His shoes were worn; his trousers were rumpled and stained; his shirt was frayed at the collar and missing most buttons at the front; his head hair was distinctly unkempt and the facial hair consisted of non-designer stubble, decorated with small pieces of rotting food. Apart from the white coat, his only credible claim to presence in the hospital at that time of night was the stethoscope in its pocket. However, its use would have necessitated insertion into the ears of two hollow metal tubes terminating in coarse screw threads because the plastic earpieces that should have been held by those threads were missing.

Mr. Porter summed up the evidence before him and concluded that the man was a vagrant with no right to be in the establishment that he was guarding, so he confronted him.

"Excuse me, sir, can I ask what you are doing in the hospital?"

"Can't you see I'm a fucking doctor?" came the swift reply.

I thought I should try a similar approach when dealing with the prison staff but felt that it would be what we in the medical profession call a bad idea.

Once the initial barrier to prison entry has been overcome, the next obstacle to negotiate is the prison timetable. More often than not, the dastardly criminal (who, of course has not yet been tried) is not currently available because he is in his cell/at work/at dinner/on exercise/in interview with probation/working on a chain gang (for all I know). Anyway, he has to be brought to the medical centre, which could take Some Time, Time That Could Have Been Avoided, the staff explain, if adequate arrangements had been made because, you see, he could have been moved In Good Time before my arrival, thereby not wasting My Valuable Time.

There are only two places in the world where time takes precedence over the job to be done. School and prison.
William Glasser

Experience teaches that this obstacle is not disastrous because the time waiting for arrival of this particular component of the criminal fraternity (who, of course has not yet been tried) is offset by the time taken in negotiating the remainder of the hazards. Often all personal belongings have to be placed in a locker at the prison entrance before one is allowed to walk from reception to the entrance to the cells. Failure to place all items, including sheets of typewritten paper, at the outset can lead to a journey back to the lockers, often a surprising distance from the cell area, because the staff are certainly not going to take the items from you or establish the innocence or otherwise of the typewritten papers by reading them.

Following this step is the removal of most of one's clothes for the X-ray screening followed by redressing without the benefit of a dressing room, table or mirror. Finally, is the Dance of the Keys. Prison warders support long chains hanging from around the area of the waist and bedecked with a multitude of shiny keys. The principle of prison is that things are locked so the warden has to have a key for practically everything. Because, I imagine, the locked items include television doors, book covers and cornflake packets, the innumerable keys required can impart a heavy toll to their porter. The resulting burden imposes on the warden the gait of a knight bedecked in hundredweights of chainmail with a pleasant musical accompaniment of one key jingling upon another.

There are usually a few hundred doors to get through to get anywhere near the vicinity of the prisoner (or so it seems) so there is ample opportunity to witness some of the more complex steps of the Dance of the Keys whereby the warden stops and pulls up the chain of keys in front of and across his body with a terminal twist of the wrist that allows the correct key to land precisely in the centre of the palm of the hand, whence the key is advanced to the lock, the whole exercise being accomplished in one uninterrupted motion.

Perhaps I shouldn't complain. Others probably have more difficulty in negotiating prisons than I do. Certainly the prisoner's friend who wants to take his mate out for a recreational break by helicopter has been effectively thwarted by the wires that crisscross above the quadrangle once serving as a makeshift heliport. And prisoners have had such difficulty with the security arrangements that at least one has been given government money to sue the prison because he became injured whilst trying to escape.

A visitor's exit from the prison is usually accomplished more easily than the entry because no appointment or identification is required. The prisoner's availability within a busy timetable is also irrelevant because they are not encouraged to accompany you. The Dance of the Keys does play its encore at exit albeit in reverse order from entry but, beyond the last security barrier, the wardens leave their visitors to their own devices, to be free, as it were, at resort.

On one occasion, the last barrier to freedom bordered onto one of the prison's quadrangles. I was gestured by the prison's representative to cross the open space, where, I was told, I would find a door that would lead me into the unrestricted wide world. As I reached the door, an exiting gentleman, whom I judged not to be a prisoner, held the door for me as I passed through. It made the sound of finality as it closed behind me. Realising that this was not the prison exit but the entrance to what appeared to be a series of offices (all locked), I reversed my route and attempted to pass through the doorway that had permitted my entrance just a few minutes earlier. On this occasion, it was considerably less yielding; in fact, it was locked.

By now, it was late afternoon in winter and darkness had descended over the prison quadrangle. As I gazed out through a window that overlooked it, I perceived that the whole establishment was heading towards a state of lockdown. Large numbers of people, presumably employees rather than inmates, were hurrying towards the exit. Guard dogs were parading the concrete yard in front of me, restrained by unusually burly prison officers. There was little doubt, even though I could not see it, that all prisoners were being returned to the cells from whatever activity had occupied them that afternoon.

I banged on the window to alert one of the exiting staff to my predicament but received, in return, a glance so filled with distrust that it reminded me instantly of the difficulty I had had in getting into the prison in the first place. A few more people behaved similarly, all quickening their step at the sight of me, staring from the adjacent window. Eventually, the institutional paranoia lifted long enough for a passer-by to recognise my plight and fetch someone else who, to my good fortune, was blessed not only with insight but also a key.

Upon my release into the quadrangle, I began to explain how I had ended up locked in an office block, when all I wanted to do was to go home but his understanding was not coupled with sympathy; in fact, he was clearly not interested. Maybe he had experienced the same problem all too often in the past; any philanthropy involved in releasing innocent victims from their misfortune had long faded; it was more fun to keep people locked up than to free them; and his pleas to the prison management to put up clear exit signs had fallen on deaf ears. To be fair, I suppose clear directions to the way out are the last things a prison needs.

Homosexuality in Russia is a crime and the punishment is seven years in prison, locked up with the other men. There is a three-year waiting list. Yakov Smirnoff

A second major reason for a doctor to be asked to see an accused is to determine whether he or she is fit to stand trial. Various medical conditions can render a person unfit but a common one for the neurologist is dementia or other form of intellectual impairment that causes the person to be disadvantaged in giving evidence in court. Failure to recall detail and difficulty in understanding and answering questions can be easily interpreted as unwillingness and lack of cooperation if no medical explanation for the behaviour can be found. Conversely, if there is such a mitigation, it indicates that the accused will not be able to give a fair account of him or herself in the witness box or be able to counter allegations made against him by others.

The most dramatic such scenarios occur when the medical state of the person becomes questionable for the first time in mid-trial because the proceedings have then to be halted until a doctor can be found to provide an assessment. By its very nature, it is an urgent matter but even more so because judges, on the whole, do not like waiting.

I was asked to see a man at as short a notice as can be imagined because it seemed evident that he was having difficulty in recounting his testimony and answering questions in the witness box. Something was likely to be wrong, I surmised, because the problem had been acknowledged by the prosecution who are notoriously cynical on such occasions. I managed to find time the next day to get down to court where

I was briefed by the defence counsel on the essentials of the case.

Dermot O'Flaherty was an Irish traveller who lived in a fixed community on the outskirts of Stoke-on-Trent near to Alton Towers theme park. He was accused of sexual assault on at least three girls, aged sixteen to eighteen years, twenty years previously. The girls claimed that they were invited into O'Flaherty's caravan to smoke his cigarettes and drink his lager and it was there that the assaults took place. One of the girls had recently had a dream in which she experienced a flashback to one such occasion. She related the contents of the dream to the other girls who instantly recalled similar mini-parties in O'Flaherty's residence, usually culminating in assault. Each time they went back, the same thing happened.

Relatively superficial enquiries had revealed that he was indeed resident in a travellers' park around that time and that the girls were also living in the area and visited several of the travellers on regular occasions. O'Flaherty could just about remember living there but easily confused it with other parks and had forgotten most of the other residents who, it was established, had been living in close proximity to him for many years. He could not remember the girls and strongly denied the allegations on the grounds that he would certainly have remembered something so important and anyway such activities were not within his nature.

In his defence, other witnesses, mostly from the same community, gave evidence that the girls were well known in the area as the self-named Gutter Grime Girls who spent most of the waking day and part of the night smoking, drinking alcohol and making use of illicit substances. These witnesses volunteered that the girls had provided sexual favours to O'Flaherty willingly, in return for booze, drugs and sometimes cash to support their lifestyle. The witnesses were all at pains to stress that similar facilities had not been provided by the girls to any of them.

I was concerned about the girls' lifestyle and their memory of the events. I raised the matter with the barrister.

"Do they admit that they were taking large quantities of drugs and alcohol during this period?"

"Yes, they do," he replied. "They admit that their way of life was not exemplary, at least as judged by society's views of the day, that compared with average behaviour patterns theirs would fall somewhat short and that many people, especially those with some degree of selfless contribution to society, would tend to look down upon them, notwithstanding that the circumstances of which we speak took place in the distant past, or relatively so, and that the same assessment made today may yield a completely different pattern of results, for the simple and so far unquestioned reason that all the girls involved with the case have, without exception, changed for the better in the years that have intervened between the events currently forming part of this legal action and the present time."

"That seems abundantly clear." I continued: "In that case, what evidence is there concerning the effects of the drugs and alcohol upon their memory for the events of that period?"

He smiled. "A good question, Dr. Sagar, in my opinion at least, my assessment of your enquiry not being influenced, I should stress, by my fortuitously having the insight to pose the very same manner of interrogation to one of the girls under cross-examination when I specifically enquired concerning the state of her memory following exposure to a number of substances that are arguably recognised to be toxic to the brain, not only by the most erudite of the medical profession, but also the majority of the lay public, thereby allowing me to raise the issue at this stage without supportive evidence, or otherwise, from a witness or witnesses with the relevant expertise in the matters that I put to you."

"What did she say?"

"What?"

"I was just asking what she said."

"That is what she said," he replied. "She said, 'What?' Accordingly, I posed the question in an even simpler form, in short enquiring of the girl the state of her memory following repeated exposure to drugs and alcohol."

"What did she say then?" I asked.

"It's fucked," he replied.

I went on to examine Dermot O'Flaherty and gave him some standardised tests of memory and other intellectual functions. It was clear that he had moderately severe dementia, probably Alzheimer's disease.

He was deemed unfit to stand trial and all legal proceedings were halted. I never did find out who was telling the truth.

One bright summer's day, when any self-respecting sun-worshipper would be prostrate in the park, clothes lifted, lowered or opened to the borderline of decency, I found myself instead sitting behind the defence barrister in Court One. The pine-boarded room boasted technological advance sufficient to communicate with involuntary prison occupants by video but not to any form of system, air conditioning or otherwise, that could reliably lower the ambient temperature. It was what we in the medical profession call hot. As I was contemplating whether the environmental conditions were designed deliberately to undermine a witness's resistance to cross-examination (i.e interrogation), my thoughts were abruptly interrupted by the sonorous voice of the court usher.

"Court rise!" Was this the latest levitation act of a part-time member of the Magic Circle designed to alleviate boredom amongst waiting lawyers, court employees and criminals? Was the courtroom and its occupants about to make a slow ascent into the clouds, to be followed by thunderous applause from the appreciative witnesses to this truly remarkable act and a beaming smile of appreciation from its executioner? No - the usher was acting like a toastmaster to announce the arrival of the next guest at the party. On this occasion, however, the introduction was much less genteel and we all knew who was coming: the judge. Everyone stood.

At a later trial, as I was again waiting for the judge to decide when he would grace us with his presence, I realised that the claimant in the case had been seriously injured and was completely dependent on a wheelchair for any form of mobility. How would the court usher announce His Lordship's arrival on this occasion? Would it be "Court rise! - except that is, for the man in the wheelchair"? And supposing there were other disabled witnesses - or even occupants of the public gallery - what would happen then? Would it be "Court rise! - except for the man in the wheelchair, the lady in green with the arthritic knees and the fat man in the grey overcoat with a bad back"? Does the clerk of the court have to do a pre-trial disability assessment on all the court attendees? Does he require special training for the purpose? I decided that the usher would be better off with an announcement that had the benefit of universal applicabilty, such as "Court rise, where possible, but no shirkers!"

Anyway, back to the trial by sauna. As usual on such occasions, the judge appeared through the side door and walked towards his seat with a gait that showed frank indifference to the courtroom and its occupants, if such a demonstration were possible. After the customary bowing, he sat down. His facial expression changed instantaneously from one of total passivity to one that well communicated a combination of boredom and intolerance. It remained so throughout the rest of the proceedings apart from occasions, which were frequent, when, no longer able to contain his frustration, he threw a minor wobbly. Civil cases, such as this one was, have no jury so the judge was the complete arbiter of the evidence presented by the barristers, one for the Claimant and one for the Defendant.

A judge is a law student who grades his own papers. Henry Louis Mencken

Counsel for the Claimant began to outline the case, which was one of medical negligence. Mrs. Carruthers, it transpired, had innocently attended an outpatient appointment at her local hospital for an opinion on her uncontrollable dandruff. Contrary to her expectations, she was not greeted by the consultant dermatologist in charge of the clinic but by "some sort of nurse" who proceeded to interrogate her not only in respect of the scalp complaint but also every other illness that she had had throughout her life and indeed many that she had not had.

Having reached this point in the story, the barrister found himself interrupted forcibly by the judge who pointed out that he had received the relevant papers in the case only the previous morning and could not guarantee to be as conversant with the contents as would perhaps be ideal. He may have to rely on Counsel to guide him through certain sections, depending upon how the evidence unravelled.

After assuring the judge that he was only too happy to assist (if, indeed, he had any choice), the barrister continued, "After the questioning, the nurse, whom we know to be Ms. Judith Lyons, took Mrs. Carruthers' temperature and pulse and then proceeded to take her blood pressure. It became obvious to Mrs. Carruthers that the nurse was having considerable difficulty because she made many attempts, each requiring inflation and deflation of the cuff around Mrs. Carruthers' upper arm. On several of these attempts, Mrs. Carruthers felt sure that the pressure in the cuff had been raised to very high levels because the sensation around her upper arm was one of intense squeezing. Furthermore, it was likely that the pressure was maintained for what we would argue was an unreasonable period because Mrs. Carruthers experienced intense throbbing in the upper arm on a number of occasions during the nurse's attempts."

"Other than the discomfort thus far described, which, we submit, was in itself not insignificant, Mrs. Carruthers felt no untoward consequences of the nurse's actions until some two weeks later, when she developed what could only be described as an intense pain spreading from the shoulder down the right arm, the one that had been involved in the nurse's attempts two weeks previously. Two days later, Mrs. Carruthers was alarmed to find that the strength in the right arm was diminishing. The weakness of the arm increased over the next few days until the arm was rendered virtually useless."

"Although the power in the arm has, to a very large extent, returned, the Claimant suffered loss of amenity related to her injuries for a period approaching six months."

"We have the benefit of expert opinion from Dr. Clinton, a consultant neurologist, who is present in court and is prepared to give evidence to the effect that Mrs. Carruthers' problems arose as a result of damage to the nerves in the arm caused by excessive pressure within the tissues of the arm and resulting directly from the wholly inadequate attempts of the nurse to take her blood pressure."

"We submit, My Lord, that the actions of Ms. Lyons were directly responsible for the injuries and consequent loss of amenity suffered by Mrs. Carruthers. Further, those actions fell short of reasonable clinical practice and were therefore negligent. Mrs. Carruthers deserves to be compensated for the negligent actions of Ms. Lyons and the disability that was thereby caused."

Law and medicine make good bedfellows. Each one looks after victims of the other.

I was there because I held a different opinion from Dr. Clinton. I believed that Mrs. Carruthers' symptoms were typical of brachial neuritis, a condition that causes inflammation of the nerves into the arm, resulting in pain and weakness. The cause is not known but it arises spontaneously and has nothing to do with the taking of blood pressure.

I had a number of reasons to disagree with Dr. Clinton: nerve damage had never previously been reported following the taking of blood pressure; the pressure produced in the arm could never be enough to damage nerves, even if the pressure were pumped up to the maximum allowed by the machine; the symptoms did not come on for two weeks whereas they should have come on immediately if the nerve were damaged at the time of the blood pressure reading; and electrical tests had shown that the site of nerve damage was further up the arm than the cuff could ever have been placed. It was also noteworthy that Dr. Clinton only ever produced reports on behalf of claimants and never defendants, a fact that might just imply a bit of bias. Defence Counsel and I had rehearsed these points to what we felt was the point of perfection and felt little doubt that we would win the case.

Eventually, Mrs. Carruthers was called to the witness box and our barrister had his turn to cross-examine.

"Mrs. Carruthers, how long after Ms. Lyons took your blood pressure did you first notice any symptoms?"

"Immediately", she replied.

"Immediately?" he said with an expression of startle that was clearly exaggerated for effect. He went on to refer to her signed statement in which she had stated that they developed after two weeks.

"So which is correct? Immediately or after two weeks?" he fired at her, adding condescendingly "Help us, Mrs. Carruthers."

"Well, both," she replied, shifting a little uneasily from side to side in the witness box. "I had problems straight away but they got worse two weeks later."

"Really?" For this question, his voice rose in pitch and became more clipped. As he spoke, his head tilted slightly to the right; he raised his eyebrows and looked her straight in the face. Already, his performance was becoming worthy of a place in the Royal Shakespeare Company.

"Did you consult your general practitioner about your symptoms during that first two weeks?" he offered, almost as an aside.

"I don't remember."

"Think hard. Help us, Mrs. Carruthers."

The judge, who, for most of the previous discourse, had been sighing and shaking his head and scribbling notes with obvious reluctance, suddenly interjected.

"Mr. Fotheringay, the witness has quite clearly indicated that she cannot remember. What is the point of pursuing this line of enquiry?"

"Your Lordship, I was attempting to establish beyond doubt that she did not attend her general practitioner because there is no record of her attendance at the surgery. Page 325 in Your Lordship's bundle refers."

The judge sighed again. "Well, she won't remember going if she didn't attend, will she?" he said with a sneer and glance at the court that seemed effectively to convey his views that the defence barrister was a total moron. "Anyway, continue" he said with another sigh before resuming his bored and intolerant demeanour.

In the courtroom of honor, the judge pounded his gavel to show that all's equal and that the courts are on the level and that the strings in the books ain't pulled and persuaded. Bob Dylan "The Lonesome Death of Hattie Carroll"

"Thank you, My Lord." Mr. Fotheringay remained remarkably composed. In fact, despite the best attempts of His Lordship to ruffle his feathers, he was probably the only one in the court room-cum-oven who was not sweating.

Later in the cross-examination, Mr. F focussed on Mrs. Carruthers' financial situation during the period of inability to use her right arm.

"You were off work for six months, Mrs. Carruthers - is that correct?"

"Yes."

"And were in receipt of a full range of benefits during that time?"

"Yes."

"Including unemployment and disability benefits?"

"Yes."

"On the understanding, of course, that you were unable to work or look after yourself. In short, you couldn't really do anything, could you?"

"No. I was completely disabled."

"Indeed," he said with a tone that conveyed complete understanding of her plight. He paused briefly and took a deep breath.

"You are normally a very active person, I understand. How did you pass your time when you were off work?" he continued nonchalantly.

"Well, there wasn't much I could do. I used to sit and read but it's not easy just using your left hand."

"No, I can see. I expect you also got lonely, didn't you? Normally you work with a lot of people; isn't that correct?"

"Yes, I do but I spent a lot of time round at my parents' place, trying to be useful."

Mr. Fotheringay paused again momentarily and then probed, "In what way?"

"I helped out with the business accounts. I read out the figures and Mum entered them onto the spreadsheet."

"How much time did you spend doing the accounts?"

"Well, it's bookkeeping really, dealing with orders, bills, income, stocks and so on, so it has to be done every week. It takes nearly two days."

"That sounds a very worthwhile thing to do and obviously helped your parents' business. I am glad you were able to occupy yourself productively." He smiled at her.

"Thank you." She smiled back.

"Did your parents pay you for your efforts?"

"Yes. We agreed on two days each week at senior secretary rates."

He paused for longer and seemingly more pointedly. With his gaze now fixed on the judge, he asked her, "Did the Benefits Office know about that?"

If barristers do not play chess, they should do because they are masters at playing the long game and drawing their opponent into a trap from which they cannot escape. Alternatively, they could be military strategists if they just had a bit more spare time.

The court is like a palace of marble; it's composed of people very hard and very polished. Jean de la Bruyère

The judge tolerated this conversation without interruption, spending most of the time motionless with his head bent forwards and to the left, as if listening carefully, pondering deeply or sleeping soundly. I wanted to believe that he had some sympathy for the points drawn out by Mr. Fotheringay which clearly implied, without of course stating, that Mrs. Carruthers was a money-grabbing opportunist who did not even play her manipulative game within the rule of law.

His Lordship decreed that we should have a lunchtime adjournment of two hours, returning to court at 2:30 p.m. Apparently the lengthy break would give him time to examine some of the key papers of the case, following a morning session that had familiarised him with the main facts. He also indicated that the day, in a court sense, would end about 4 p.m. but there should be ample time in the afternoon session for Dr. Clinton to give his evidence.

Dr. Clinton walked briskly and confidently to the witness box with a thick file of papers held under his left armpit. He stood erect, with his hands clasped loosely in front of him and head slightly extended. He declined the offer from the judge to take a seat. He obviously meant business.

After Dr. Clinton had given his evidence-in-chief, guided by the gentle and almost obsequious questioning of Counsel for the Claimant, Mr. Fotheringay rose for his cross-examination.

"Dr. Clinton, the essence of your analysis of this case, as I see it, is that Mrs. Carruthers sustained damage to the nerve or nerves in the arm as a result of pressure applied to the nerve from the inflated blood pressure cuff." The pause that followed was terminated after a few nanoseconds by His Tetchy Lordship:

"Is that a question, Mr. Fotheringay?"

"Well, Your Lordship, inasmuch as I am inviting Dr. Clinton to agree or disagree, the answer to your question must be 'yes.'"

The judge turned towards Dr. Clinton. "You are being asked whether you agree or disagree."

"I agree," said Dr. Clinton with deliberation.

"Continue," said the judge, returning to his notes.

"Thank you, Your Lordship," said Counsel. "Dr. Clinton, do you know the magnitude of the pressure that is required to induce nerve damage?"

With a slight smirk, Dr. Clinton turned towards the judge and said, "I am afraid I am a simple doctor, not a bioengineer, so I cannot answer that question with any expertise." The judge nodded.

"Are you aware of any situations where pressure can cause nerve damage?" asked Counsel.

"Oh yes," effused Dr. Clinton. "Pressure from a tumour can do it and, of course, the optic nerve is damaged by raised pressure in the eye in glaucoma. Those are just two examples."

"I trust you will agree that, in those cases, the pressure is applied over a much longer period than would occur during the taking of Mrs. Carruthers' blood pressure."

"The risk of damage depends on two factors: the intensity of the pressure and its duration," replied Dr. Clinton.

"Precisely so," said Mr. Fotheringay. "Perhaps I should put the question more simply."

"That would be helpful," interjected the judge.

"Have you ever seen, heard of or read about nerve damage resulting from the taking of someone's blood pressure?" continued Mr. F.

"No, but many things reported for the first time are hailed as great discoveries," observed Dr. Clinton.

"Are you saying that your observations in this case represent one of those 'great discoveries'?" enquired Mr. Fotheringay.

"No, I am simply saying that, because it has not been observed previously, does not mean it is incorrect."

Mr. Fotheringay changed tack. "May I draw your attention to the neurophysiological tests? My understanding is that these are essentially electrical tests that measure how well the nerves conduct. Is that understanding correct?" Mr. F probably knew enough about neurophysiological tests to write his own textbook but was also an arch protagonist of the "Softly, softly, catchee monkey" approach, at least as applied to law.

"Yes," replied Dr. Clinton.

"Again, my understanding - and please, Dr. Clinton, correct me if that understanding is misguided - is that these studies showed the site of nerve damage to be further up the arm than any blood pressure cuff could reasonably have been placed."

Mr. F was slowly creeping up on his prey.

"Do you agree with that interpretation and, if so, could you please assist the Court by explaining how those findings are consistent with nerve damage produced by a blood pressure cuff?" continued Counsel. By now, any bodily movement had ceased and he was staring straight towards Dr. Clinton who, by contrast, was looking downwards through half-closed lids with his mouth slightly open. Suddenly, Dr. Clinton looked up, closed his mouth and turned towards the judge.

"Yes, thank you. I think, My Lord, that swelling in the tissues of the upper arm caused by obstruction to blood flow in the veins must have led to extension of the damage further up the arm."

Counsel quickly turned around to me and whispered "Is that correct? Does that happen?"

"No," I replied simply.

Mr. Fotheringay turned back to Dr. Clinton. "Can you provide any evidence in support of that suggestion?" he asked with just a hint of a snap.

Dr. Clinton beamed. "Only thirty years of clinical experience." That is the sort of answer produced by old hands at the expert-witness game when trapped into a corner because it is impossible for a barrister to contradict, short of claiming outright that the doctor's professional career has been fundamentally misguided, and who would want to claim the authority to be able to make that suggestion to someone from a different profession?   Instead, he sighed heavily, an unspoken indication to the judge to take account of the doctor's well-recognised ruse. The judge showed no reaction.

Mr. F continued with his questioning. "You will have heard Mrs. Carruthers giving her evidence when she stated that the symptoms deteriorated two weeks after their onset. How do you explain that when the general rule is that symptoms tend to be maximal immediately after a traumatic event? Do you agree with that general rule?"

"Yes, as a generalisation," replied Dr. Clinton, almost deliberately unhelpfully, it seemed.

"And in Mrs. Carruthers' case?"

"I interpret the deterioration as a reflection of inflammation that developed in the tissues after the trauma," he said, nodding towards the judge, who was not looking.

"Can I assume it is again clinical experience that leads you to that conclusion?"

"Yes."

"Are you aware of any scientific evidence in support of your observations?" This was about as far as Mr. F dare go as a challenge to Dr. Clinton's authority without appearing unprofessional himself.

"Surprisingly, there is little published on these mechanisms," said Dr. Clinton.

I did not attend the next day when the two barristers each summed up their case but the solicitor, who was present, told me that Mr. Fotheringay had reiterated with clarity the key objections to the claim that the nerve damage was caused by the blood pressure cuff and had submitted to the judge that Dr. Clinton's explanations to those objections were his honest belief but had no objective evidence to support them. Much more likely, he said, was that Mrs. Carruthers had suffered an episode of brachial neuritis. This was a well-recognised condition and her symptoms were typical of it. Its onset had nothing to do with the taking of her blood pressure.

His Lordship, in expressing his judgement, had spoken well of both expert witnesses. He was, however, alarmed at the apparent increase in accidents and illnesses caused by medical misdemeanour and recommended that the government review urgently the efficacy of existing procedures to safeguard the general public. He had enormous sympathy for Mrs. Carruthers because six months of her life had been blighted by her disability. Although recognising the difficulties in interpretation of the evidence, he indicated that not to find in her favour would deprive her of compensation for the consequences of somebody else's actions, a situation that would be wholly unacceptable.

I think that meant that he believed the story about the blood pressure cuff but it's hard to tell. Anyway, she won.

This is a court of law young man, not a court of justice. Oliver Wendell Holmes

All of Rubin's cards were marked in advance. The trial was a pig-circus, he never had a chance. Bob Dylan "Hurricane"

Medical negligence cases, more than others, mostly fall into two diametrically opposed categories: those that are nonsense claims and those that are obviously indefensible. The nonsense cases commonly arise because treatment fails to produce complete recovery, an outcome that is understandably distressing for the sufferer. Unfortunately, nature is not allowed to be an influential force in these situations and the failure of the patient to return to normal following their illness is translated by them as "somebody's fault". There is also an underappreciation that medical intervention, whether by medication or by surgery, is potentially risky and complications can still occur, even though everyone involved in the therapy has behaved in an exemplary fashion. Life is hazardous, after all; in fact, it is ultimately and universally fatal.

Some people think that doctors and nurses can put scrambled eggs back in the shell. Cass Canfield

It is, of course, important to tell the patient of potential risks because, by law, consent to treatment has to be "informed". To avoid the risk of litigation, some consultants will go to heroic lengths to ensure that the patient has all the necessary information, speaking to them in one-to-one minilectures and handing out reams of information sheets.

We might yet hear, "Because we are operating upon your spine, there is a risk that we will damage the spinal cord. Depending upon the extent of this damage, you may develop problems with your arms and legs. In the worst case scenario, you will be completely paralysed and have total loss of sensation below the neck. You may also lose control of your bladder so you will need a permanent catheter and become sexually impotent. In addition, there is always a risk of infection developing within the site of the operation. In theory, this could spread and you could develop septicaemia, otherwise known as blood poisoning. Obviously, that is a serious condition and indeed can be fatal. If bleeding occurs during the surgery or afterwards, you may need a blood transfusion. These days, donors' blood is carefully screened but, of course, it is always possible that you would contract hepatitis or AIDS from it."

A carefully judged administration of scare tactics may lead the patient to decline the operation completely on the grounds that there seems a lot to accept just to get rid of some pain in the neck. The benefit to the surgeon would be that failure to operate removes completely any risk of being sued, frees up space in the operating theatre and thereby reduces the waiting list for surgery, much to the glee of the hospital managers.

You can die of the cure before you die of the illness. Michael Landon

One day, I received a large package containing a solicitor's letter of instruction and a bundle of medical records. This event, in itself, did not surprise me because receipt of large volumes of paper, courtesy of Britain's lawyers, had, by now, become commonplace. Indeed, at one point, I had considered moving house in order to accommodate all these communiques until I discovered the services of professional shredders. But the content of the papers was surprising, at least when I finally got round to reading them (sometimes the world of law moves inexorably slowly and it's easy to catch the habit).

Instructing solicitors told me that they represented the defendant in a claim for alleged medical negligence. The claimant had been involved in a road traffic accident, causing personal injury. He continued to have physical disability as a result of that accident, despite attendance at hospital during the immediate aftermath of the accident. They claimed, on his behalf, that delay in his treatment was directly responsible for his continuing problems. The defendant admitted treating the claimant in the Accident and Emergency Department but did not believe that there was any delay, given the circumstances of the case. Furthermore, even if there had been a delay, he did not believe that the patient had suffered in any significant way as a result of it.

My first, possibly prejudicial reaction, was that here was another case of a poor patient, who had suffered at the hands of the motorist, seeking to transfer the cause of that suffering to the hands of the doctor or, even worse, was someone trying to maximise his compensation by suing both parties. On reading the notes, I fully expected to read of a person who had suffered a minor whiplash neck injury in a rear shunting collision, had not recovered fully and blamed the fifteen-minute wait in the Accident and Emergency Department for all life's woes, or at least those that followed the road accident.

Not so. It did not take long to find out that this was a serious case. For a start, the most recent summary from the home rehabilitation service described him as "still dependent on a wheelchair" and "has to be assisted in all daily tasks because of persisting severe weakness of the arms". He had a mechanical aid to collect his urine into a leg bag because he had no awareness of when or how to pass urine.

I delved further into the medical records. After review of a few hundred pages, most of which were, as usual, irrelevant, I felt I had built up a reasonable picture of the case. Mr. Bennett had sustained brain damage at birth which had left him with severe epilepsy and balance difficulties so he was looked after in a care home. He was able to get about on his own, albeit with some difficulty, but his carers chose to move him in a wheelchair when outdoors for safety reasons.

The irony of this reasoning was established on the day of the accident when Mr. Bennett's excursion in the fresh air was abruptly interrupted by a collision between his wheelchair and a passing car. Mr. Bennett was being pushed across the road by his carer with a green light in his favour but sadly the car pursuing a route across his path was driven by someone who seemed not to understand that different-coloured traffic lights conveyed different instructions or who suffered from severe red-green colour blindness. Mr. Bennett was thrown from his wheelchair but the carer following by necessity a little behind avoided the ensuing impact.

Both Mr. Bennett and his carer were taken to hospital where he received an assessment of his physical injuries and she received treatment for psychological trauma, comprising a hot cup of tea, a seat and enquiry as to whether she would be able to cope on her own or needed the nursing staff to contact a close and understanding relative.

After a few hours, it was decided to allow both of them home with a decision that Mr. Bennett did not need any follow-up appointment because his cuts and bruises would heal of their own accord. His carer was told that she should return for an urgent specialist consultation if her distress at witnessing a potentially serious and certainly frightening accident did not improve within a few days.

Unfortunately, once back at the care home, it became clear that all was not well with Mr. Bennett. Specifically, he could no longer walk. The carer who had accompanied him to hospital had, by this time, gone home early with emotional distress but the other workers in the home felt that they could manage without the benefit of her detailed account of the previous few hours. They contacted the Accident and Emergency Department and were advised that they should bring Mr. Bennett back to hospital if he had not improved by the following day. With some difficulty because of his inability to cooperate, they finally managed to get him into bed where he slept until the next morning.

On finding that he was no better and indeed appeared to be worse in so far as he could now move neither his legs nor his arms, his carers bundled him into a car and returned him to hospital. Just before they left, his carer from the scene of the accident telephoned to say that her doctor had given her three weeks' sick leave for emotional trauma but she felt it might not be enough, particularly after learning of that morning's developments.

On this occasion, Mr. Bennett was investigated by X-rays which showed a fracture of a vertebra in the neck and sliding of one vertebra over another. A CT scan of the neck showed that the spinal cord had been compressed and had visible signs of trauma at the level of the neck. In essence, he had broken his neck in the accident; the neck had become unstable; and, as a result, the spinal cord had been damaged. The main nerves to the arms and legs pass through the spinal cord at that level so Mr. Bennett had sustained paralysis of his arms and legs as a result of the neurological damage. He never recovered but the good news is that his carer was eventually able to return to work.

At the case conference a few months later, the barrister explained:

"The critical issues in this case - if I may put it that way, bearing in mind that I am not referring to the critical medical matters, essential though they are to any issue arising outside the medical context, but to the key legal points - are: firstly, whether or not the spinal injury was a direct result of the accident, a point which I imagine is not too contentious; secondly, whether the injury should reasonably have been detected by the examining doctor in the Accident and Emergency Department; thirdly, whether the chosen course of his management would reasonably have been different if such a detection were forthcoming; and, fourthly, whether any damage, over and above that resulting from the accident itself, has resulted from not having followed such a course, bearing in mind specifically that the injured gentleman was allowed to return to his normal domicile with, as far as we can assess - and do correct me if you have evidence to the contrary from the medical records or elsewhere - no advice concerning activities to avoid, if there be any, supervision or happenings that may reasonably precipitate a return to the Accident and Emergency Department by the patient under consideration, with or without the assistance of others, who most obviously in his case would be his carers. Is that clear, Dr. Sagar?"

"Abundantly," I replied. All in a single sentence again - these guys are beyond belief, I thought.

I continued, "Well, we know that the examining doctor was aware something was wrong because he wrote in the notes that Mr. Bennett was unable to walk and that was a new development. He recorded that the reflexes in the legs were abnormally brisk. He should have suspected a spinal injury and arranged X-ray of the neck. He wrongly sent him home. Because the neck was unstable, it is very likely that Mr. Bennett sustained additional damage to the spinal cord during the period before he was readmitted."

"Thank you for your succinctness" said the barrister "a quality which, I have to admit, I sometimes find lacking in the accounts and explanations of expert witnesses, and, for that matter, non-expert witnesses as well, not, of course, I should add hastily, intending to make by this comment any generalisation that could be applied without consideration to each and every member of the profession or trade to which the criticism be applied or to which one may even consider application of such criticism."

"No, indeed."

We rapidly established that the actions of the doctor were, yes, negligent, yes, grossly negligent and, yes, indefensible. However, the barrister still managed to spin out the conference for two hours. Barristers' conferences always last two hours.

The journey back to the hospital was in one of those downpours that require a windscreen wiper speed so fast that it would almost certainly induce heart failure in a proportionate human activity. The mist rising from the road and the darkening skies restricted visibility to a level not much better than that of my smog-filled journeys home from school through central Manchester in the 1960s. Perhaps it was this melancholic environment that induced my introspective ruminations on The System. By the time of my arrival at the *Krankenhaus,* where I could resume my primary role of healing the sick, I had formulated a number of conclusions:

Doctors are practitioners of medicine, highly trained and at great expense, who sometimes make mistakes.

Solicitors and barristers are practitioners of law, highly trained and at great expense, who sometimes make mistakes.

Criminals and incompetents occur in all walks of life.

Legal cases are decided by competition between two opposing sides.

The nature and extent of available medical services are often decided by competition between different specialities.

Self-interest is a powerful motivator.
Would that it were not so.

By the old wooden stove where our hats was hung,
Our words were told, our songs were sung
Where we longed for nothin' and were quite satisfied
Talkin' and a-jokin' about the world outside.....
..........Ten thousand dollars at the drop of a hat
I'd give it all gladly if our lives could be like that.
Bob Dylan "Bob Dylan's Dream"

Chapter 11: Postscript

The Wednesday General Neurology Clinic had gone like every one before it: a cross-section of society passing through its doors over the space of three to four hours and displaying a representative sample of conditions from any standard neurological textbook. The usual percentage of patients had failed to attend; one turned up with no appointment booked for that day and three arrived late. Of those three, one had telephoned to say they were held up in traffic; one had tried but could get no answer from the hospital switchboard; and one had not bothered. One lady had got angry and another cried.

I had five telephone calls during the clinic: one from a consultant in orthopaedics asking me to see one of his patients on the ward; another from a GP asking me to do a domiciliary visit in Hexthorpe when I was next in Doncaster; a third from a solicitor asking me to hurry up with the report on one of their clients; a fourth from my secretary telling me that the Medical Staff Committee meeting at 5 p.m. had been cancelled because the chairman had been suddenly called away; and the last from my wife asking me to buy Easy-garlic and one tin each of Italian tomatoes and chopped onions on the way home for a spaghetti bolognese recipe from the Simply Cooking series of her monthly Women At Home magazine.

I was able to deal with some patients well within the allotted time but significantly more required longer than allowed. Taking into account the effect of the telephone interruptions, the result was that the clinic was, as usual, running late.

It was a normal day. Bob Dylan "Talking World War III Blues"

The last patient of the morning came into my room at 1:15 p.m., thirty minutes later than her scheduled appointment. She was in her thirties, well dressed with long black hair and an elfin face. She wore scarlet lipstick. She was in a wheelchair.

I had first seen her ten years earlier when she was working as an accountant. She presented then with a bout of double vision and dizziness that cleared completely over a few weeks but she later had further symptoms and, by now, her multiple sclerosis was badly disabling.

"I am sorry to keep you waiting Miss Sanderson," I said, "but we have had one or two problems this morning. How are you?"

"I'm great. In fact, I'm having a ball - even though I can't really do anything. Life's a barrel of laughs." And she did indeed laugh.

"It's really nice to see you in good spirits."

"I'm sure Doctor that, like me, you've been around doctors, hospitals, patients and all the rest that medicine has to offer long enough to know that sometimes, as far as your experience is concerned, if you didn't laugh, you'd cry."

"How true."

Tolling for the aching ones whose wounds cannot be nursed, for the confused, accused, misused, strung-out ones and worse, and for every hung-up person in the whole wide universe. And we gazed upon the chimes of freedom flashing. Bob Dylan "Chimes of Freedom"

It's all right, Ma. It's life and life only. Bob Dylan. "It's All Right Ma; I'm Only Bleeding"

Printed in Great Britain
by Amazon